D0535364

light meals with meat

microwave cooking library®

by barbara methven

microwave cooking library®

If you want to eat light and eat right, try meat. Think of the variety you can enjoy by adding beef, pork, lamb and veal to the menu. You don't have to compromise your low-fat, low-cholesterol life-style. *Light Meals with Meat* shows you how to choose and cook "skinny" cuts—the ones with no more than 3 grams of fat per ounce and fewer than 200 calories in a 3-ounce serving. Recipes feature fresh ingredients and reduced fat and sodium products for healthy, balanced meals that rate low in fat and high in flavor and eating enjoyment. See for yourself how food that is good for you can also taste terrific. Designed for healthy people who want to stay healthy, *Light Meals with Meat* helps you "eat fit" and eat meat, too.

Barbara Methven

Barbara Methven

CREDITS:
Design & Production: Cy DeCosse Incorporated
Art Directors: Yelena Konrardy, David Schelitzche
Project Director: Peggy Ramette
Project Manager: Deborah Bialik
Home Economists: Ellen Meis, Kristin K. Moss, Peggy Ramette, Ann Stuart, Grace Wells
Dietitian: Hill Nutrition Associates, Inc.
Consultants: Susan Lamb Parenti, Dianne R. McCroskey Phillips, Joanne Randen
Editors: Janice Cauley, Bernice Maehren
Director of Development Planning & Production: Jim Bindas
Production Manager: Amelia Merz
Electronic Publishing Analyst: Joe Fahey
Production Staff: Adam Esco, Peter Gloege, Melissa Grabanski, Eva Hansen, Jeff Hickman, Jim Huntley, Mark Jacobson, Daniel Meyers, Mike Schauer, Linda Schloegel, Greg Wallace, Nik Wogstad
Studio Managers: Rebecca Boyle, Cathleen Shannon, Rena Tassone
Lead Photographers: John Lauenstein, Mark Macemon
Photographers: Rex Irmen, Mette Nielsen, Mike Parker, Cathleen Shannon
Contributing Photographers: Dave Brus, Linda Glantz, Charles Nields
Food Stylists: Sue Brue, Bobbette Destiche, Darcy Gorris, Nancy Johnson
Contributing Food Stylists: Mara Crombie, Christine Gruidl, Melinda Hutchison, Robin Krause, Kathy Lightly, Amy Printy, Madelin Streu, Cindy Syme
Color Separations: Scantrans
Printing: R. R. Donnelley & Sons (1191)

Additional volumes in the Microwave Cooking Library series are available from the publisher:

- Basic Microwaving
- Recipe Conversion for Microwave
- Microwaving Meats
- Microwave Baking & Desserts
- Microwaving Meals in 30 Minutes
- Microwaving on a Diet
- Microwaving Fruits & Vegetables
- Microwaving Convenience Foods
- Microwaving for Holidays & Parties
- Microwaving for One & Two
- The Microwave & Freezer
- 101 Microwaving Secrets
- Microwaving Light & Healthy
- Microwaving Poultry & Seafood
- Microwaving America's Favorites
- Microwaving Fast & Easy Main Dishes
- More Microwaving Secrets
- Microwaving Light Meals & Snacks
- Holiday Microwave Ideas
- Easy Microwave Menus
- Low-fat Microwave Meals
- Cool Quick Summer Microwaving
- Ground Beef Microwave Meals
- Microwave Speed Meals
- One Pound of Imagination: Main Dishes
- One-dish Meals

CY DE COSSE INCORPORATED
Chairman: Cy DeCosse
President: James B. Maus
Executive Vice President: William B. Jones

Library of Congress Cataloging-in-Publication Data

Methven, Barbara
  Light Meals with Meat / by Barbara Methven.

  p.   cm. — (Microwave cooking library)
Includes index.
ISBN 0-86573-573-5

  1. Microwave cookery 2. Cookery (Meat) I. Title. II. Series.
TX832.M3938   1992   91-42438
641.6'6 — dc20

Copyright © 1992 by Cy DeCosse Incorporated
5900 Green Oak Drive
Minnetonka, MN 55343
1-800-328-3895
All rights reserved
Printed in U.S.A.

Approved by the Beef Industry Council, Pork Industry Group, Lamb Committee, and Veal Committee of the National Livestock and Meat Board, and reviewed by the National Pork Producers Council.

Contents

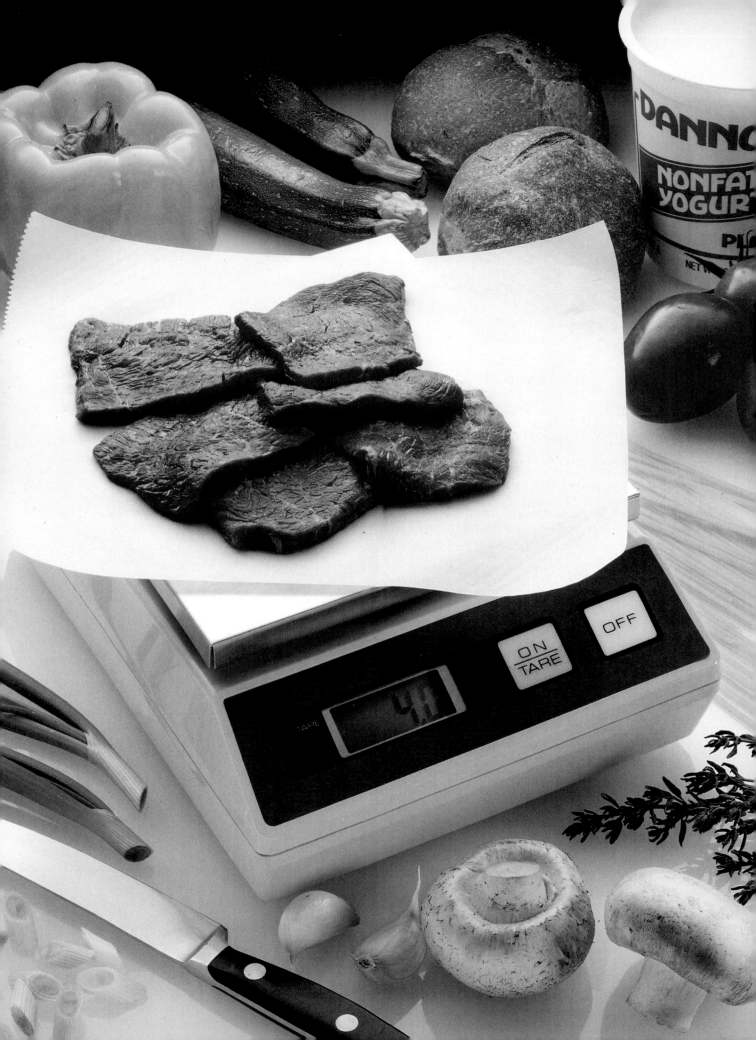

What You Need to Know Before You Start

If you and your family are suffering from "chicken fatigue," the good news is that you can eat meat and still eat light by choosing the leaner cuts, which compare favorably in nutrition with poultry and fish, and provide welcome variety.

The "skinny" cuts of meat featured in this book contain no more than 10 grams of fat per *3-ounce* cooked portion and 200 or fewer calories per serving. *Light Meals with Meat* shows you how to select and use lean cuts of meat to put variety and flavor back into your light meals.

What is light?

This is not a diet book. It's for healthy people who want to stay healthy. It provides a menu style you can live with, long term. These light maintenance meals contain no more than 22 grams of fat, including accompaniments. They are based on the USDA recommendation of no more than 30% calories from fat and a limit of 2000 calories per day.

What is a meal?

A good, healthy meal is balanced, and that means variety. It includes meat, vegetables, fruit, starch and dairy products. The entrée recipes in this book, with the serving suggestions, provide complete nutrition.

That can't be light!

Eating light and right with meat doesn't mean deprivation. These fresh, flavorful meals make a few fat calories count. With a touch of olive oil or a dollop of lean sour cream, they use limited fats for flavor, not just to grease a pan and prevent sticking.

The cooking method may be grilling, microwaving, roasting, braising or stir-frying. For each cut of meat, we recommend the right method to keep lean meats low-fat, tender and juicy.

Don't defeat the purpose of your light meal by lavishing margarine or butter on your low-fat dinner roll, or smothering a salad with rich dressing. Choose low-fat dressings or spreads, and use about half as much as you normally use.

How to Use This Book

Each of the three main sections includes recipes for beef, pork, lamb and veal. Individual servings of cooked, trimmed meat provide *3-ounce* portions. The charts on pages 8 to 13 picture the skinny cuts and provide nutritional data.

Recipes for boneless cuts allow *4 ounces* of un-cooked, trimmed meat per serving. Weights for bone-in cuts vary, depending on the amount of bone. An 8-ounce bone-in trimmed pork chop will yield 3 ounces of cooked meat, while a serving of lamb chops starts with two 5¾-ounce-each uncooked, bone-in trimmed chops.

Fast & Flavorful. Prepare these meals from start to finish in 30 minutes or less. No recipe has more than eight ingredients. For a fresh, contemporary approach to meat cookery, some recipes feature fresh vegetables and fruits, as well as less familiar ingredients, like roasted red peppers or pesto.

Enlightened Old Favorites. Serve your family's traditional favorites, like pot roast or chili. To fit today's healthy eating style, these recipes reduce fat calories and keep old-fashioned flavor.

Hot off the Grill. Learn how to grill skinny cuts of meat and keep them tender and juicy. Directions include traditional grilling and micro-grilling—a techinique for precooking some meats and vegetables to speed up final grilling. Recipes include multipurpose marinades and grilled accompaniments as well as entrées.

Nutritional Information

Per-serving nutritional values and exchanges for weight loss follow each recipe. When a recipe serves four to six persons, the analysis applies to the greater number of servings. In the case of alternate ingredients, the analysis applies to the first ingredient listed. Optional ingredients are not included in the analysis. When a recipe calls for a marinade that will be drained and discarded after use, the analysis allows for partial absorption. If a portion of the marinade is set aside for sauce or is used in the recipe prior to the addition of meat, the nutritional values for that amount are calculated separately.

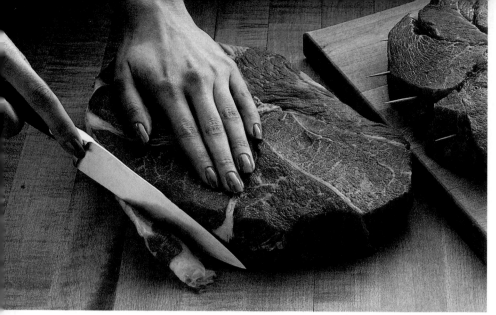

Keeping Lean Meat Lean

On the following pages, you will find charts for lean cuts of beef, pork, lamb and veal (including pictures to help you identify them), and recommended cooking methods. Once you have selected a skinny cut of meat, don't spoil the result by adding unnecessary fat during cooking. A little attention will preserve the benefits of lean cuts of meat.

Trim fat before cooking. Most meat cutters market well-trimmed leaner cuts. However, an individual meat cut may benefit from judicious trimming at home. If you cut out a piece of intermuscular fat, skewer the meat with a wooden pick to maintain a compact shape during cooking.

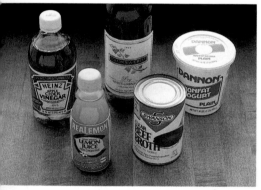

Reduce oil in marinades. Acidic foods, such as lemon juice, vinegar, wine or yogurt, tenderize the meat. You can substitute water or broth for all or part of the oil.

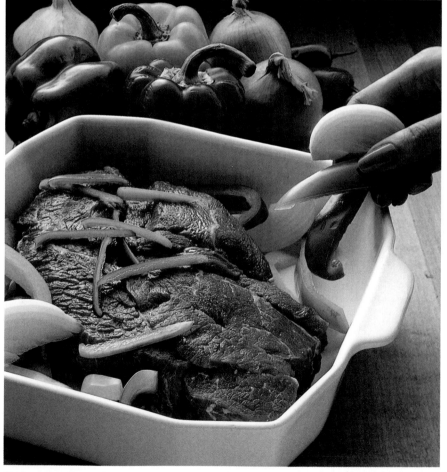

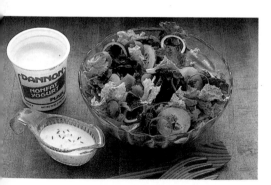

Make low-fat substitutions. Use yogurt instead of mayonnaise in salad dressings and replace sour cream with light sour cream in sauces.

Enhance flavor with fresh ingredients. Green or red peppers, onions, garlic, ginger or chilies contribute flavor without adding fat, sugar or salt.

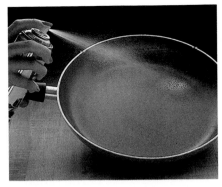

Treat cooking surfaces with nonstick spray. Don't add extra fat to your lean meat by searing or sautéing it in oil, margarine or butter.

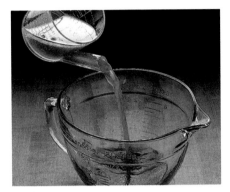

Skim fat from broth or sauce. To skim fat from hot liquid, put liquid in a skimmer cup, which allows you to pour off the liquid while the fat remains in the cup. Another way is to chill liquid until fat hardens so you can skim it off the surface.

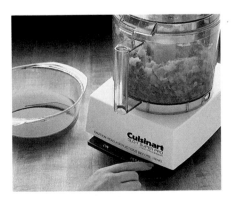

Lighten sauces. Purée cooked vegetables, like onions, carrots, potatoes or legumes, to give body to sauces, soups and stews; or thicken sauces with cornstarch instead of flour (1 tablespoon thickens 1 cup liquid).

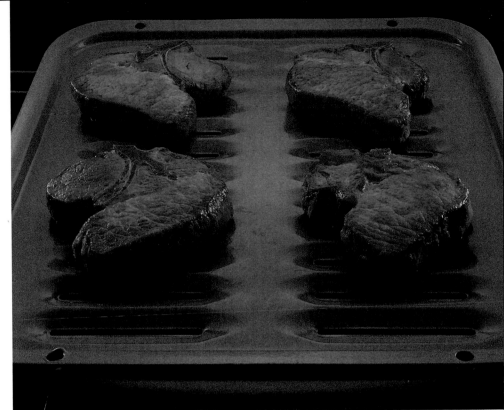

Broil meat on a rack. The drip pan catches any fat rendered from the meat, while the rack keeps fat from clinging to the meat's surface.

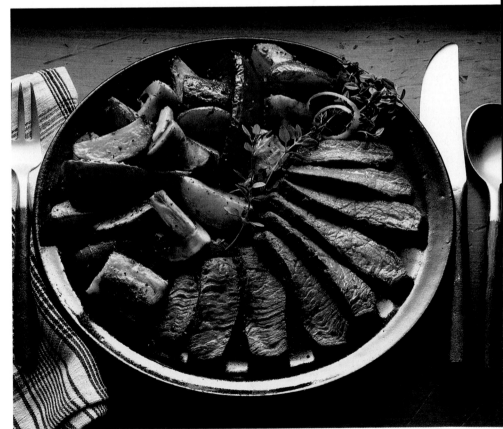

Carve meats before serving. In a single piece, a 3-ounce portion of meat may look skimpy to someone not used to eating light. When sliced and fanned out on the plate, it looks like a more substantial serving. Also, some cuts are easier to eat when carved thinly across the grain.

Skinny Cuts (Beef)

Tender	Cooking Method	Nutritional Information
Sirloin Steak	Oven Roast, Broil, Grill, Panbroil, Microwave (Strips)	Per 3-oz. roasted, trimmed portion: *Calories: 165* *Protein: 26 g.* *Fat: 6 g. (2 g. saturated fatty acids)* *Cholesterol: 76 mg.*
Tenderloin Roast Steaks	Roast: Oven Roast, Grill Steak: Broil, Grill, Panbroil, Microwave	Per 3-oz. broiled, trimmed portion: *Calories: 179* *Protein: 24 g.* *Fat: 9 g. (3 g. saturated fatty acids)* *Cholesterol: 71 mg.*
Top Loin (Strip Steak) Steak	Oven Roast, Broil, Grill, Panbroil	Per 3-oz. broiled, trimmed portion: *Calories: 176* *Protein: 24 g.* *Fat: 8 g. (3 g. saturated fatty acids)* *Cholesterol: 65 mg.*

Intermediate Tender	Cooking Method	Nutritional Information
Round Tip Roast Steak	Roast: Oven Roast Steak: Broil, or Grill when Marinated, Panbroil Thin-cut Steaks	Per 3-oz. roasted, trimmed portion: *Calories: 157* *Protein: 24 g.* *Fat: 6 g. (2 g. saturated fatty acids)* *Cholesterol: 69 mg.*
Top Round Roast Steak	Roast: Oven Roast Steak: Broil, or Grill when Marinated, Stir-fry, Microwave (Strips)	Per 3-oz. broiled, trimmed portion: *Calories: 153* *Protein: 27 g.* *Fat: 4 g. (1 g. saturated fatty acids)* *Cholesterol: 71 mg.*

Intermediate Tender (continued)	Cooking Method	Nutritional Information
Eye Round Roast Steak	Roast: Oven Roast, or Butterfly and Broil Steak: Broil, or Grill when Marinated	Per 3-oz. roasted, trimmed portion: *Calories: 143* *Protein: 25 g.* *Fat: 4 g. (2 g. saturated fatty acids)* *Cholesterol: 59 mg.*
Chuck Shoulder (Arm) Roast Steak	Roast: Braise Steak: Braise or Broil, or Grill when Marinated	Per 3-oz. braised, trimmed portion: *Calories: 183* *Protein: 28 g.* *Fat: 7 g. (3 g. saturated fatty acids)* *Cholesterol: 86 mg.*
Flank Steak	Broil or Grill when Marinated, Stir-fry	Per 3-oz. broiled, trimmed portion: *Calories: 176* *Protein: 23 g.* *Fat: 9 g. (4 g. saturated fatty acids)* *Cholesterol: 57 mg.*
Less Tender	**Cooking Method**	**Nutritional Information**
Bottom Round Roast	Roast: Braise Cubed Steaks: Panbroil	Per 3-oz. braised, trimmed portion: *Calories: 178* *Protein: 27 g.* *Fat: 7 g. (2 g. saturated fatty acids)* *Cholesterol: 82 mg.*
Shank Crosscuts	Braise, Cook in Liquid	Per 3-oz. braised, trimmed portion: *Calories: 171* *Protein: 29 g.* *Fat: 5 g. (2 g. saturated fatty acids)* *Cholesterol: 66 mg.*

Skinny Cuts (Pork)

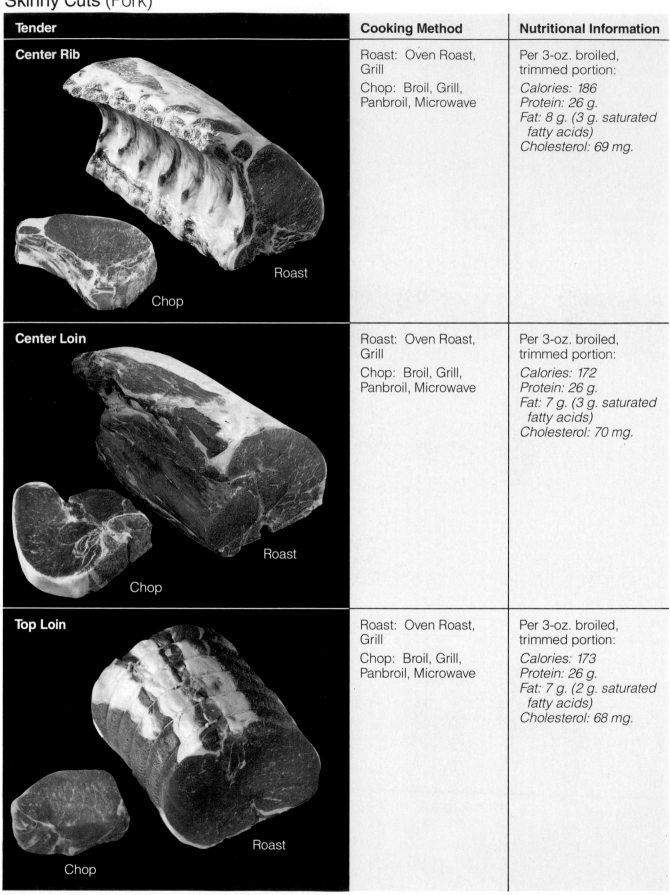

Tender	Cooking Method	Nutritional Information
Center Rib — Roast, Chop	Roast: Oven Roast, Grill Chop: Broil, Grill, Panbroil, Microwave	Per 3-oz. broiled, trimmed portion: *Calories: 186* *Protein: 26 g.* *Fat: 8 g. (3 g. saturated fatty acids)* *Cholesterol: 69 mg.*
Center Loin — Roast, Chop	Roast: Oven Roast, Grill Chop: Broil, Grill, Panbroil, Microwave	Per 3-oz. broiled, trimmed portion: *Calories: 172* *Protein: 26 g.* *Fat: 7 g. (3 g. saturated fatty acids)* *Cholesterol: 70 mg.*
Top Loin — Roast, Chop	Roast: Oven Roast, Grill Chop: Broil, Grill, Panbroil, Microwave	Per 3-oz. broiled, trimmed portion: *Calories: 173* *Protein: 26 g.* *Fat: 7 g. (2 g. saturated fatty acids)* *Cholesterol: 68 mg.*

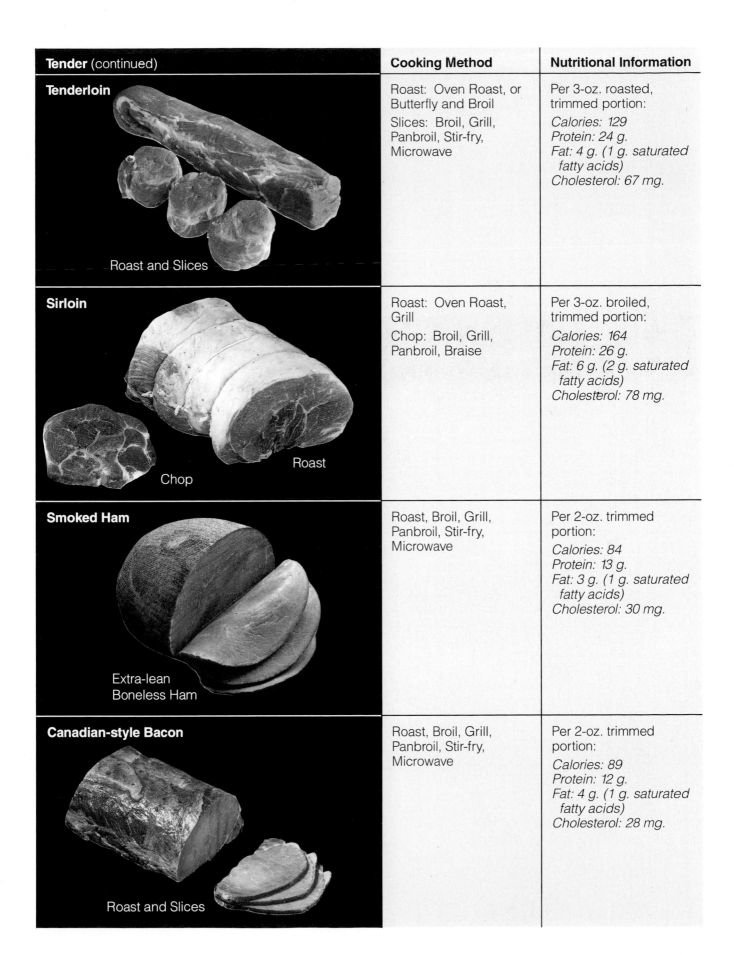

Tender (continued)	**Cooking Method**	**Nutritional Information**
Tenderloin Roast and Slices	Roast: Oven Roast, or Butterfly and Broil Slices: Broil, Grill, Panbroil, Stir-fry, Microwave	Per 3-oz. roasted, trimmed portion: *Calories: 129* *Protein: 24 g.* *Fat: 4 g. (1 g. saturated fatty acids)* *Cholesterol: 67 mg.*
Sirloin Chop Roast	Roast: Oven Roast, Grill Chop: Broil, Grill, Panbroil, Braise	Per 3-oz. broiled, trimmed portion: *Calories: 164* *Protein: 26 g.* *Fat: 6 g. (2 g. saturated fatty acids)* *Cholesterol: 78 mg.*
Smoked Ham Extra-lean Boneless Ham	Roast, Broil, Grill, Panbroil, Stir-fry, Microwave	Per 2-oz. trimmed portion: *Calories: 84* *Protein: 13 g.* *Fat: 3 g. (1 g. saturated fatty acids)* *Cholesterol: 30 mg.*
Canadian-style Bacon Roast and Slices	Roast, Broil, Grill, Panbroil, Stir-fry, Microwave	Per 2-oz. trimmed portion: *Calories: 89* *Protein: 12 g.* *Fat: 4 g. (1 g. saturated fatty acids)* *Cholesterol: 28 mg.*

Skinny Cuts (Lamb & Veal)

Lamb — Tender	Cooking Method	Nutritional Information
Shoulder Blade Chop Roast	Chop: Braise or Grill, or Broil when Marinated Roast: Braise or Oven Roast	Per 3-oz. broiled, trimmed portion: *Calories: 179* *Protein: 22 g.* *Fat: 10 g. (3 g. saturated fatty acids)* *Cholesterol: 78 mg.*
Leg Roast	Oven Roast, Grill or Broil when Butterflied	Per 3-oz. roasted, trimmed portion: *Calories: 162* *Protein: 24 g.* *Fat: 7 g. (2 g. saturated fatty acids)* *Cholesterol: 76 mg.*
Rib Chop Roast	Chop: Broil, Grill, Panbroil Roast: Oven Roast or Grill	Per 3-oz. roasted, trimmed portion: *Calories: 197* *Protein: 22 g.* *Fat: 11 g. (4 g. saturated fatty acids)* *Cholesterol: 74 mg.*
Loin Chop Roast	Chop: Broil, Grill, Panbroil Roast: Oven Roast or Grill	Per 3-oz. broiled, trimmed portion: *Calories: 183* *Protein: 25 g.* *Fat: 8 g. (3 g. saturated fatty acids)* *Cholesterol: 80 mg.*

Lamb — Less Tender	Cooking Method	Nutritional Information
Shank Whole	Braise, Cook in Liquid	Per 3-oz. braised, trimmed portion: *Calories: 159* *Protein: 26 g.* *Fat: 5 g. (2 g. saturated fatty acids)* *Cholesterol: 89 mg.*

Veal — Tender	Cooking Method	Nutritional Information
Leg Cutlet	Panfry, Panbroil, Braise, Stir-fry	Per 3-oz. panfried, trimmed portion: *Calories: 156* *Protein: 28 g.* *Fat: 4 g. (1 g. saturated fatty acids)* *Cholesterol: 91 mg.*

Veal — **Tender** (continued)	Cooking Method	Nutritional Information
Loin Chop	Oven Roast, Broil, Grill, Panbroil	Per 3-oz. roasted, trimmed portion: *Calories: 149* *Protein: 22 g.* *Fat: 6 g. (2 g. saturated fatty acids)* *Cholesterol: 90 mg.*
Rib Chop	Oven Roast, Broil, Grill, Panbroil	Per 3-oz. roasted, trimmed portion: *Calories: 151* *Protein: 22 g.* *Fat: 6 g. (2 g. saturated fatty acids)* *Cholesterol: 97 mg.*
Veal — Intermediate Tender	**Cooking Method**	**Nutritional Information**
Shoulder Steak Roast	Steak: Broil, or Grill when Marinated Roast: Braise	Per 3-oz. roasted, trimmed portion: *Calories: 144* *Protein: 22 g.* *Fat: 6 g. (2 g. saturated fatty acids)* *Cholesterol: 97 mg.*
Rump Roast	Oven Roast, Braise	Per 3-oz. roasted, trimmed portion: *Calories: 128* *Protein: 24 g.* *Fat: 3 g. (1 g. saturated fatty acids)* *Cholesterol: 88 mg.*
Veal — Less Tender	**Cooking Method**	**Nutritional Information**
Shank Crosscuts	Braise, Cook in Liquid	Per 3-oz. cooked, trimmed portion: *Calories: 156* *Protein: 28 g.* *Fat: 4 g. (1 g. saturated fatty acids)* *Cholesterol: 91 mg.*
Round Steak	Braise	Per 3-oz. cooked, trimmed portion: *Calories: 156* *Protein: 28 g.* *Fat: 4 g. (1 g. saturated fatty acids)* *Cholesterol: 91 mg.*

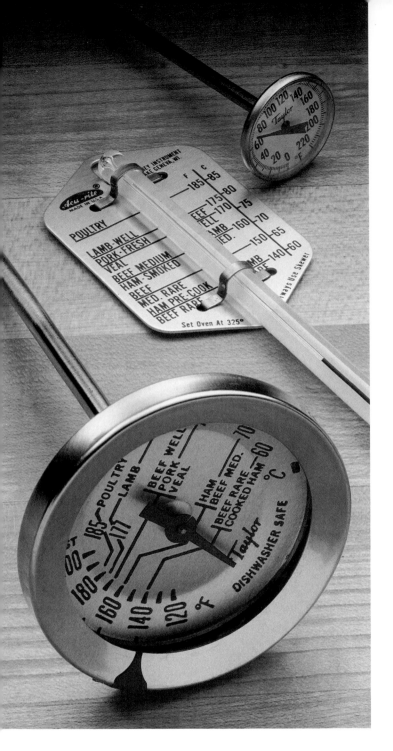

Testing for Doneness

Accurate doneness is important for leaner cuts of meat. Overcooking dries out natural juices. Doneness is less critical with fatty cuts, which may be perceived as juicy because the fat lubricates the meat even when juices have dried. Some lean cuts of beef, such as round or flank steak, may not be suitable for cooking to well done. Today's leaner pork is also sensitive to overcooking.

To be sure results are tender and juicy, use the cuts of meat recommended in the recipes and in the charts on pages 8 to 13. Test for doneness, especially when the recipe calls for a check before the addition of other ingredients or for standing time after cooking is completed.

Visual Test

Judge doneness of small cuts, such as strips, cubes, medallions, steaks or chops, by looking at them. To check, make a small slit in the center of a piece of meat.

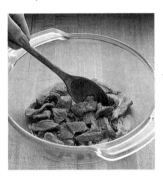

Cook beef and lamb just until meat is only slightly pink.

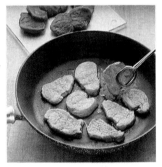

Cook pork and veal just until meat is no longer pink on the exterior, but slightly pink on the inside.

Internal Temperature

For larger cuts of meat, such as roasts, the most accurate test for doneness is internal temperature. The chart (opposite) gives recommended final temperatures. During standing time, the internal temperature of most roasts will rise 5°F. Large roasts, weighing 6 to 8 pounds, will rise about 10°F. To avoid overcooking, remove roasts from the oven, grill or microwave before the internal temperature reaches the desired doneness.

Dial and flat meat thermometers are used for large roasts. The dial thermometer has a doneness indicator that can be preset 5° to 10°F below

the desired doneness to allow for standing time. Insert these thermometers in the roast before cooking and leave them in place while the roast is in the conventional oven or on the grill. Do not use these thermometers in the microwave oven.

A rapid-response or instant-read thermometer may be used with large or small roasts. To check doneness during cooking, insert the thermometer in the meat just long enough to test the temperature, and then remove it. Do not leave the thermometer in the conventional or microwave oven.

Thermometer Check

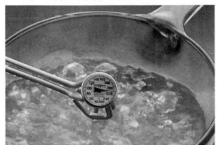

Check the accuracy of your thermometer after several years of use. If your thermometer will register as high as 220°F, place the stem in boiling water to a depth of 2 inches. It should register 212°F.

How to Insert a Thermometer

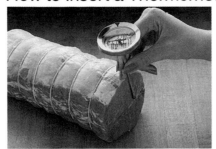

Measure the distance from the outside of the roast to the center of the thickest muscle. With your fingers, mark the point where the thermometer touches the edge of the meat.

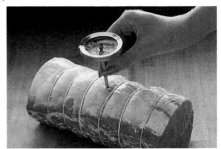

Insert thermometer to the depth marked by your fingers. Tip should be in center of meat, not touching fat or bone. With a flat roast, insert the thermometer into the end so that at least 2 inches of the stem is in the meat.

Internal Temperature Chart

Beef & Lamb

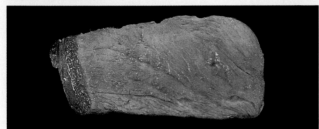

Rare 140°F: Remove roast from oven at 135°F. During standing, roast continues to cook and internal temperature rises to 140°F.

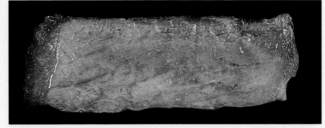

Medium-rare 150°F: Remove roast from oven at 140° to 145°F. During standing, roast continues to cook and internal temperature rises to 145° or 150°F.

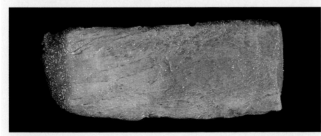

Medium 160°F: Remove roast from oven at 155°F. During standing, roast continues to cook and internal temperature rises to 160°F.

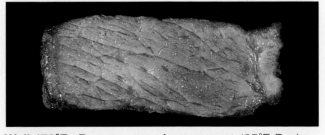

Well 170°F: Remove roast from oven at 165°F. During standing, roast continues to cook and internal temperature rises to 170°F. This degree of doneness is not recommended for intermediate tender or less tender cuts of meat.

Pork

Medium 160°F: Remove roast from oven at 155°F. During standing, roast continues to cook and internal temperature rises to 160°F. This doneness is recommended for conventional cooking only.

Well 170°F: Remove roast from oven at 165°F. During standing, roast continues to cook and internal temperature rises to 170°F. This doneness is recommended for conventional and microwave cooking.

Veal

Medium 160°F: Remove roast from oven at 155°F. During standing, roast continues to cook and internal temperature rises to 160°F.

Well 170°F: Remove roast from oven at 165°F. During standing, roast continues to cook and internal temperature rises to 170°F.

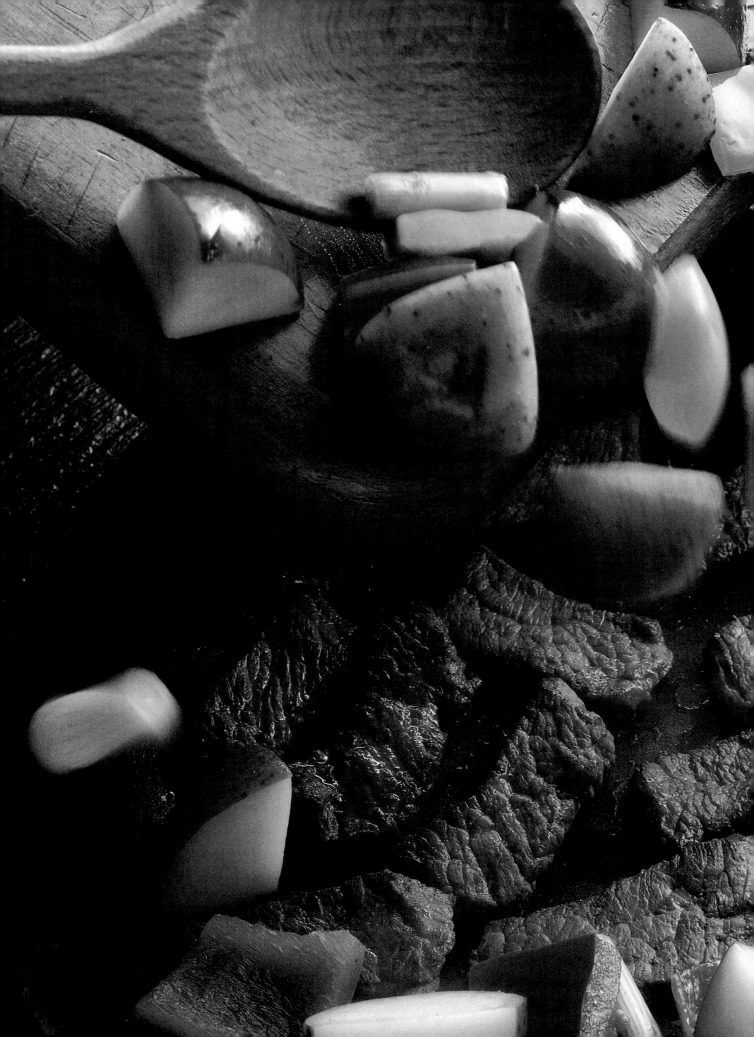

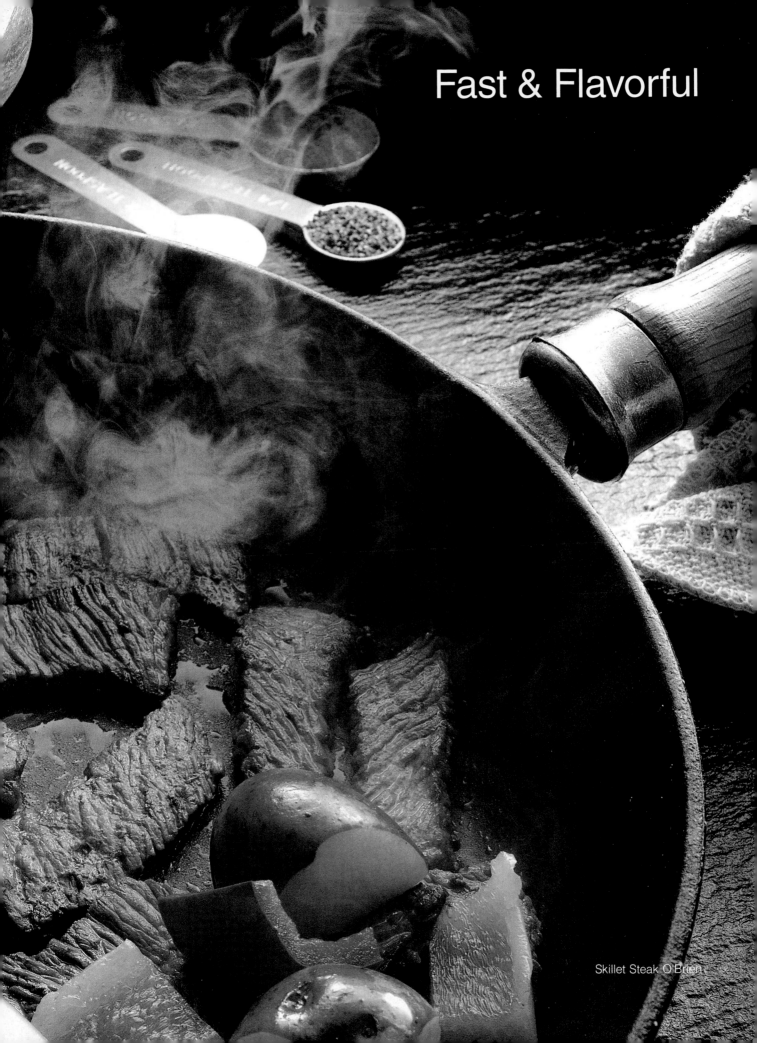

Fast & Flavorful

Skillet Steak O'Brien

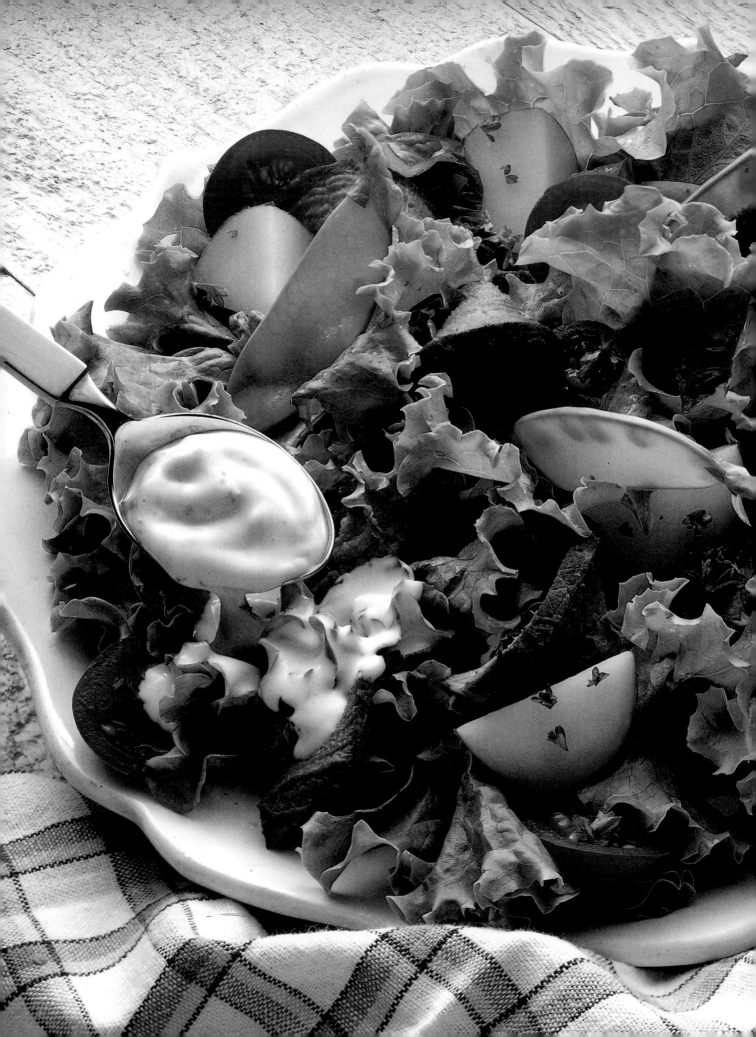

Beef

◄ Ranch Beef Salad

4 beef eye round steaks
   (4 oz. each), ¾ inch thick
¼ teaspoon onion powder
10 small new potatoes, cut
   into quarters (about 1 lb.)
2 tablespoons water
6 oz. fresh snow pea pods
   (2 cups)
   Leaf lettuce leaves
1 cup halved cherry tomatoes
⅓ cup low-fat ranch dressing
1 teaspoon snipped fresh
   parsley

4 servings

Pound steaks to ½-inch thickness. Sprinkle both sides of steaks evenly with onion powder. Spray 10-inch nonstick skillet with nonstick vegetable cooking spray. Heat skillet conventionally over medium-high heat. Cook steaks for 4 to 5 minutes, or until desired doneness, turning over once. Cover to keep warm. Set aside.

Place potatoes and water in 2-quart casserole. Cover. Microwave at High for 5 to 11 minutes, or until tender, stirring once. Drain. Remove from casserole. Set aside. In same casserole, place pea pods. Cover. Microwave at High for 2 to 4 minutes, or just until tender-crisp, stirring once. Arrange lettuce leaves on 12-inch serving platter. Carve steaks into thin slices. Arrange steak, potatoes, pea pods and tomatoes over lettuce. Drizzle dressing evenly over salad. Sprinkle with parsley.

Serving suggestion: Serve with sliced French bread or crisp bread sticks.

Per Serving: Calories: 299 • Protein: 28 g. • Carbohydrate: 26 g. • Fat: 9 g.
• Cholesterol: 65 mg. • Sodium: 237 mg.
Exchanges: 1⅓ starch, 3 lean meat, 1 vegetable

Warm Steak Salad

8 baguette slices
½ cup plus 2 tablespoons
   nonfat Italian dressing,
   divided
1-lb. well-trimmed beef top
   sirloin steak, 1 inch thick
1 teaspoon steak seasoning
6 cups torn mixed greens
   (Bibb lettuce, leaf lettuce,
   radicchio and spinach)
16 cherry or pear tomatoes

4 servings

Heat conventional oven to 350°F. Brush both sides of baguette slices lightly with 2 tablespoons dressing. Arrange in even layer on baking sheet. Bake for 8 to 10 minutes, or until golden brown, turning over once. Set aside.

Sprinkle both sides of steak evenly with steak seasoning. Place steak on rack in broiler pan. Place under conventional broiler, with surface of meat 3 to 4 inches from heat. Broil for 13 to 15 minutes, or until desired doneness, turning over once. Carve steak into thin slices. Set aside.

In 1-cup measure, microwave remaining ½ cup dressing at High for 2 to 3 minutes, or until hot. Arrange greens evenly on 4 individual serving plates. Arrange tomatoes, baguette slices and steak evenly on plates. Spoon 2 tablespoons warm dressing over each salad.

Serving suggestion: Serve with steamed green beans.

Per Serving: Calories: 293 • Protein: 30 g. • Carbohydrate: 23 g. • Fat: 7 g.
• Cholesterol: 77 mg. • Sodium: 1050 mg.
Exchanges: 1 starch, 3 lean meat, 1½ vegetable

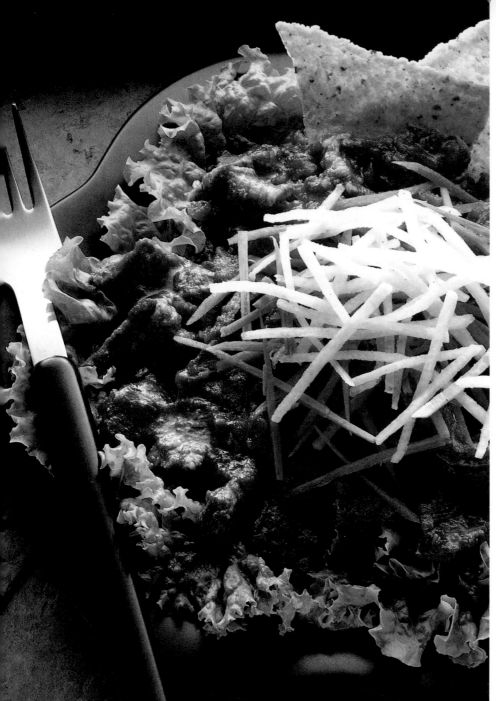

◄ Easy Beef Ensalada

    1 - lb. well-trimmed beef
        top sirloin steak, 1 inch
        thick, cut into 2 × ¼-inch-
        thick strips
    1   clove garlic, minced
    1   teaspoon ground cumin
    1½ cups salsa
    4   cups torn leaf lettuce
    ½   cup shredded carrot
    ½   cup shredded jicama
    8   tortilla chips

                            4 servings

In 2-quart casserole, combine
beef strips, garlic and cumin.
Microwave at High for 5 to 7 minutes, or just until meat is only
slightly pink, stirring once. Drain.
Add salsa to meat in casserole.
Mix well. Arrange lettuce evenly
on 4 individual serving plates.
Top evenly with meat mixture.
Sprinkle evenly with shredded
carrot and jicama. Garnish each
salad with 2 tortilla chips.

Serving suggestion: Serve with
warm corn bread.

Per Serving: Calories: 234 • Protein: 27 g.
• Carbohydrate: 14 g. • Fat: 7 g.
• Cholesterol: 76 mg. • Sodium: 634 mg.
Exchanges: ¼ starch, 3 lean meat,
2 vegetable

Creamy Beef & Basil Salad

    8   oz. uncooked rotini
    1 - lb. well-trimmed beef
        top sirloin steak, 1 inch
        thick, cut into 2 × ½-inch-
        thick strips
    1   cup frozen corn
    1½ cups halved cherry tomatoes
    ¾   cup plain nonfat yogurt
    ½   cup chopped red onion
    ½   cup snipped fresh basil
        leaves
    ¼   teaspoon salt

                            4 servings

Prepare rotini as directed on package. Rinse and drain. Set aside.
In 2-quart casserole, microwave beef strips at High for 6 to 8 minutes, or just until meat is only slightly pink, stirring twice. Drain. Set
aside. Place corn in large mixing bowl. Cover with plastic wrap. Microwave at High for 2 to 3 minutes, or until defrosted, stirring once. Rinse
with cold water. Drain. Return to mixing bowl. Add rotini, meat and
remaining ingredients. Toss to combine.

Serving suggestion: Serve with fresh melon slices.

Per Serving: Calories: 456 • Protein: 38 g. • Carbohydrate: 59 g. • Fat: 8 g.
• Cholesterol: 77 mg. • Sodium: 233 mg.
Exchanges: 3 starch, 3 lean meat, 1 vegetable, ½ skim milk

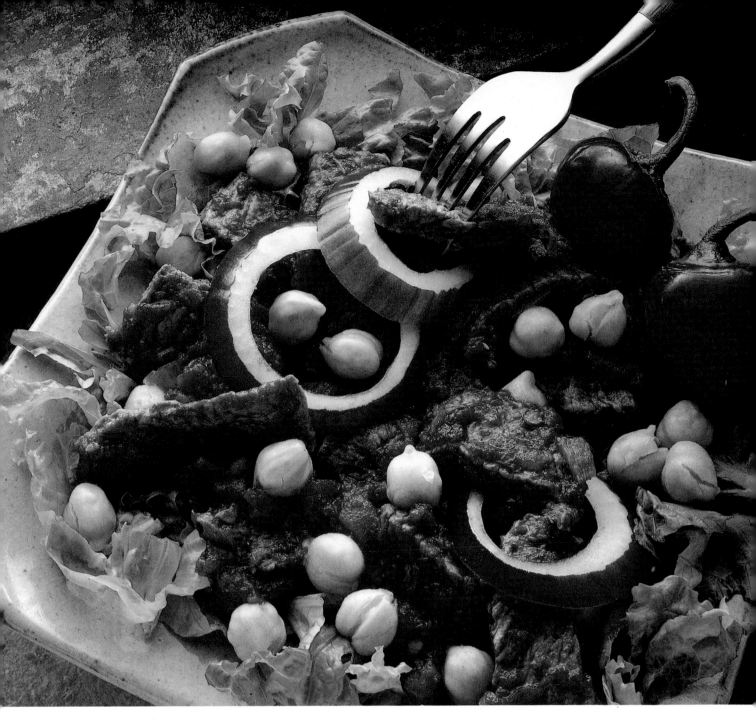

Lime Salsa Beef Salad

1 - lb. well-trimmed beef top
    sirloin steak, 1 inch thick,
    cut into 2 × ⅛-inch-thick
    strips
¾ cup salsa
1 tablespoon fresh lime juice
4 cups shredded lettuce
½ cup sliced red onion
1 cup canned garbanzo
    beans, rinsed and drained
8 sweet cherry or banana
    pickles

4 servings

Place beef strips in 2-quart casserole. Cover. Microwave at High for 5 to 7 minutes, or just until meat is only slightly pink, stirring once or twice. Drain. Stir in salsa and juice. Re-cover. Microwave at High for 2 to 3 minutes, or until hot, stirring once. Arrange lettuce evenly on 4 individual serving plates. Top evenly with meat mixture, onion, beans and pickles. Sprinkle with additional fresh lime juice, if desired.

Serving suggestion: Serve with warmed, rolled-up flour tortillas.

Per Serving: Calories: 231 • Protein: 23 g. • Carbohydrate: 24 g. • Fat: 5 g.
• Cholesterol: 52 mg. • Sodium: 515 mg.
Exchanges: 1 starch, 3 lean meat, 1 vegetable, ¼ fruit

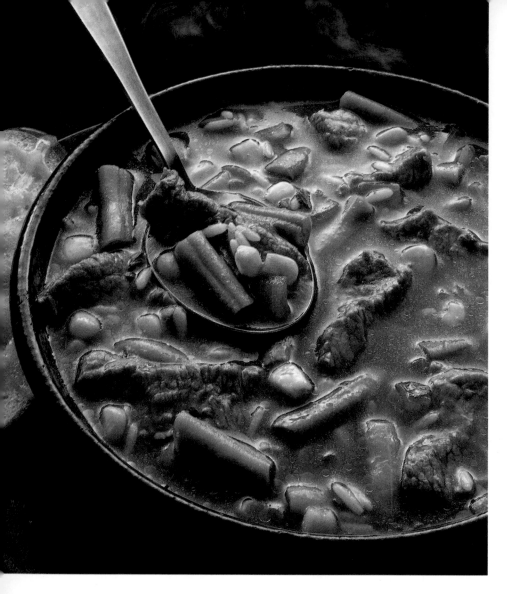

Chunky Beef & Vegetable Soup ▲

1 - lb. well-trimmed beef top
   round steak, 1/2 to 3/4 inch
   thick, cut across grain into
   1 1/2 × 1/4-inch-thick strips
1 pkg. (9 oz.) frozen green
   beans
1 cup frozen corn

1/2 cup chopped onion
2 cups tomato and chili
   cocktail
1 cup water
1/2 teaspoon dried oregano
   leaves
1/2 cup uncooked instant rice

4 servings

In 3-quart casserole, microwave beef strips at High for 5 to 7 minutes, or just until meat is only slightly pink, stirring once or twice.
Drain. Remove meat from casserole. Set aside. Add green beans,
corn and onion to same casserole. Cover. Microwave at High for 7
to 10 minutes, or until vegetables are hot and onion is tender. Add
remaining ingredients, except rice and meat. Re-cover. Microwave
at High for 7 to 11 minutes, or until beans are tender-crisp and liquid is very hot, stirring once. Stir in rice and meat. Re-cover. Let
stand for 5 minutes.

Serving suggestion: Serve with garlic toast with melted cheese.

Per Serving: Calories: 287 • Protein: 31 g. • Carbohydrate: 30 g. • Fat: 5 g.
• Cholesterol: 72 mg. • Sodium: 434 mg.
Exchanges: N/A

Old-fashioned Beef & Barley Salad

1 cup uncooked quick
   pearled barley
2 cups frozen mixed
   vegetables
1/4 cup water
1 - lb. well-trimmed beef
   top round steak, 1/2 to
   3/4 inch thick, cut across
   grain into 1 1/2 × 1/4-inch-
   thick strips
3/4 teaspoon dried thyme
   leaves, divided
1/4 cup plus 2 tablespoons
   fresh lemon juice
3 tablespoons olive oil
1/2 to 3/4 teaspoon salt

4 servings

Prepare barley as directed on
package. Rinse and drain. Place
barley in large mixing bowl or
salad bowl. Set aside. In 2-quart
casserole, combine vegetables
and water. Cover. Microwave at
High for 6 to 7 minutes, or until
vegetables are defrosted, stirring once. Drain. Add vegetables
to barley. In same 2-quart casserole, combine beef strips and
1/4 teaspoon thyme. Microwave
at High for 5 to 7 minutes, or just
until meat is only slightly pink,
stirring once. Drain. Add meat
to barley mixture. In 1-cup measure, combine juice, oil, salt and
remaining 1/2 teaspoon thyme.
Add to barley mixture. Toss to
coat. Garnish with tomato
wedges, if desired.

Serving suggestion: Serve with
Armenian cracker bread.

Per Serving: Calories: 442 • Protein: 34 g.
• Carbohydrate: 42 g. • Fat: 15 g.
• Cholesterol: 71 mg. • Sodium: 441 mg.
Exchanges: 2½ starch, 3 lean meat,
1 vegetable, 1 fat

Jamaican Beef ▶
& Pepper Pot Soup*

1- lb. well-trimmed beef top
   round steak, 1/2 to 3/4 inch
   thick, cut across grain into
   1 1/2 × 1/4-inch-thick strips
1 cup red and green pepper
   chunks (1-inch chunks)
1 can (4 oz.) chopped green
   chilies
1/2 teaspoon freshly ground
   black pepper
1/4 teaspoon ground cinnamon
1 can (28 oz.) whole tomatoes,
   undrained and cut up
1 can (14 1/2 oz.) ready-to-serve
   chicken broth
1/2 cup uncooked instant rice

4 servings

In 2-quart casserole, combine
beef strips, pepper chunks,
chilies, pepper and cinnamon.
Microwave at High, uncovered,
for 5 to 7 minutes, or just until
meat is only slightly pink, stirring
twice. Set aside. In 3-quart casserole, combine tomatoes and broth.
Cover. Microwave at High for 9
to 12 minutes, or just until mixture
begins to boil. Add meat mixture
and rice. Re-cover. Microwave
at High for 2 to 3 minutes, or
until hot. Let stand, covered, for
5 minutes.

Serving suggestion: Serve with
crusty hard rolls and fresh fruit.

*Recipe not recommended for
ovens with less than 600 cooking
watts.

Per Serving: Calories: 256 • Protein: 30 g.
• Carbohydrate: 22 g. • Fat: 5 g.
• Cholesterol: 65 mg. • Sodium: 1004 mg.
Exchanges: 2/3 starch, 3 lean meat,
2 1/2 vegetable

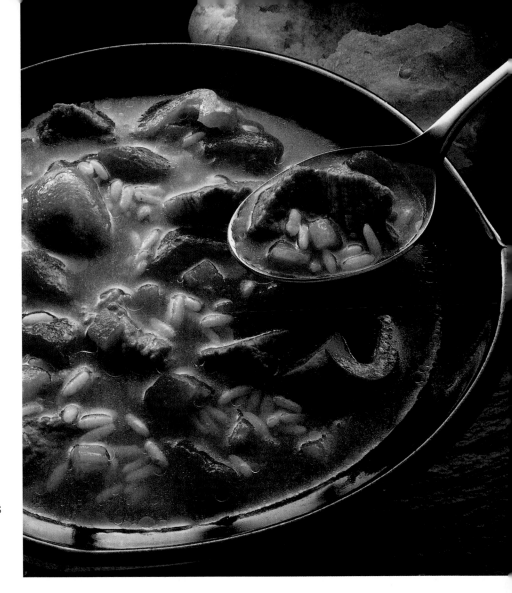

Chili with Corn & Salsa

1- lb. well-trimmed beef top
   round steak, 1/2 to 3/4 inch
   thick, cut across grain into
   2 × 1/2-inch-thick strips
1 jar (16 oz.) salsa
1 can (15 oz.) kidney beans,
   rinsed and drained

1 can (14 1/2 oz.) diced
   tomatoes, undrained
1 cup sliced green onions
1 cup frozen corn
2 teaspoons chili powder

4 servings

In 3-quart casserole, microwave beef strips at High for 6 to 8 minutes, or just until meat is only slightly pink, stirring twice. Drain. Add
remaining ingredients to meat in casserole. Mix well. Cover. Microwave at High for 15 to 17 minutes, or until onions are tender and
mixture is hot, stirring once or twice.

Serving suggestion: Serve with tortilla chips or warmed, rolled-up
flour tortillas.

Per Serving: Calories: 348 • Protein: 39 g. • Carbohydrate: 35 g. • Fat: 6 g.
• Cholesterol: 77 mg. • Sodium: 1073 mg.
Exchanges: 1 3/4 starch, 3 lean meat, 1 1/2 vegetable

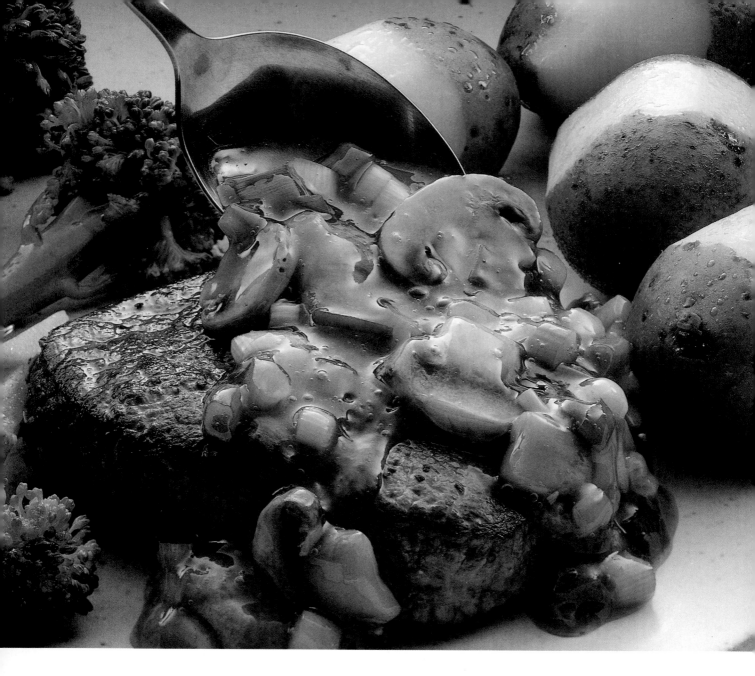

Brandy Pepper Steaks

4 beef eye round steaks
   (4 oz. each), ¾ inch thick
¼ teaspoon freshly ground
   pepper
½ cup sliced green onions
2 teaspoons cornstarch
½ cup ready-to-serve beef
   broth
4 oz. fresh mushrooms, sliced
   (1 cup)
1 tablespoon brandy

4 servings

Pound steaks to ½-inch thickness. Sprinkle both sides of steaks evenly with pepper. Set aside. In 4-cup measure, microwave onions at High for 1 to 2 minutes, or until tender. Stir in cornstarch. Blend in broth until mixture is smooth. Microwave at High for 1½ to 2 minutes, or until mixture is thickened and translucent, stirring once. Stir in mushrooms and brandy. Microwave at High for 2 to 3 minutes, or until mushrooms are tender. Cover with plastic wrap. Set aside. Spray 10-inch nonstick skillet with nonstick vegetable cooking spray. Heat skillet conventionally over medium-high heat. Cook steaks for 4 to 5 minutes, or until desired doneness, turning over once. Spoon sauce over steaks.

Serving suggestion: Serve with boiled new potatoes and steamed broccoli spears.

Per Serving: Calories: 176 • Protein: 26 g. • Carbohydrate: 3 g. • Fat: 5 g.
• Cholesterol: 61 mg. • Sodium: 165 mg.
Exchanges: 3 lean meat, ¾ vegetable

Skillet Steak O'Brien ▶

10 small new potatoes, cut into quarters (about 1 lb.)
1½ cups green and red pepper chunks (1-inch chunks)
¼ cup water
1- lb. well-trimmed boneless beef sirloin steak, 1 inch thick, cut into 2 × ¼-inch-thick strips
4 green onions, cut into 1-inch lengths (½ cup)
1 teaspoon paprika
½ teaspoon salt
¼ to ½ teaspoon pepper

4 servings

In 2-quart casserole, combine potatoes, pepper chunks and water. Cover. Microwave at High for 8 to 12 minutes, or until potatoes are tender, stirring twice. Drain. Set aside. Spray 12-inch nonstick skillet with nonstick vegetable cooking spray. Heat skillet conventionally over medium-high heat. Add beef strips. Cook for 4 to 6 minutes, or just until meat is only slightly pink, stirring frequently. Add potato mixture and remaining ingredients. Cook for 4 to 5 minutes, or until potatoes begin to brown and mixture is hot, stirring frequently.

Serving suggestion: Serve with tossed green salad.

Per Serving: Calories: 256 • Protein: 27 g. • Carbohydrate: 24 g. • Fat: 6 g. • Cholesterol: 69 mg. • Sodium: 350 mg. Exchanges: 1¼ starch, 3 lean meat, 1 vegetable

Dijon Vegetables & Flank Steak

1- lb. well-trimmed beef flank steak, cut across grain into 2 × ⅛-inch-thick strips
2 medium russet potatoes, peeled and thinly sliced (2 cups)
1 cup carrot strips (1 × ¼-inch strips)
1 cup small fresh broccoli flowerets
¼ cup plain low-fat yogurt
2 tablespoons Dijon mustard
½ teaspoon dried dill weed
⅛ teaspoon pepper

4 servings

In 2-quart casserole, microwave beef strips at High for 5 to 7 minutes, or just until meat is only slightly pink, stirring twice. Drain. Remove meat from casserole. Set aside. In same casserole, combine potatoes, carrots and broccoli. Cover. Microwave at High for 8 to 9 minutes, or until vegetables are tender, stirring twice. Add meat. Re-cover. Microwave at High for 1 to 2 minutes, or until hot. In small mixing bowl, combine yogurt, mustard, dill weed and pepper. Add to meat mixture. Stir gently to coat.

Serving suggestion: Serve with sliced fresh fruit and French bread.

Per Serving: Calories: 268 • Protein: 26 g. • Carbohydrate: 18 g. • Fat: 10 g. • Cholesterol: 58 mg. • Sodium: 328 mg. Exchanges: ⅔ starch, 3 lean meat, 1½ vegetable

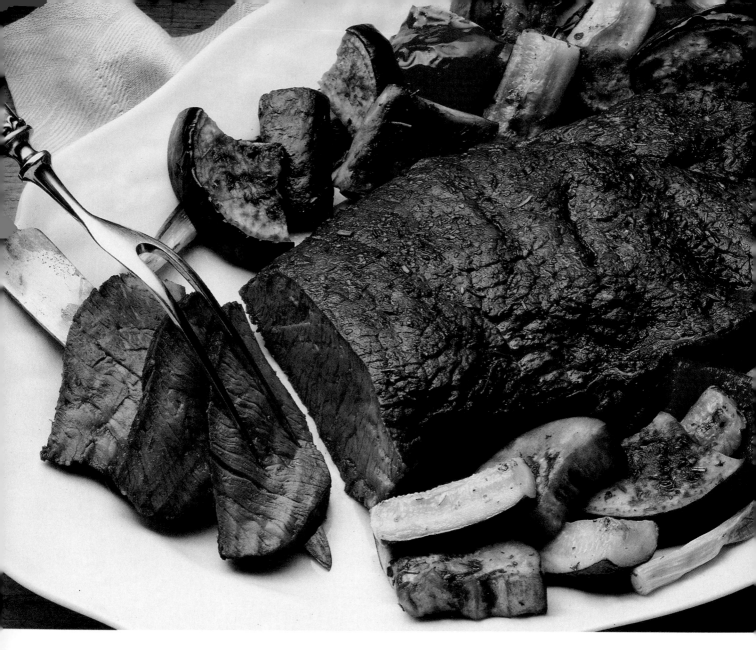

Broiled Steak & Ratatouille Vegetables

1 teaspoon Italian seasoning
½ teaspoon seasoned salt
1 - lb. well-trimmed beef top
    sirloin steak, 1 inch thick
1 medium eggplant (1 lb.),
    cut lengthwise into quarters,
    then crosswise into ½-inch-
    thick slices
1 medium red pepper, cut
    into 1½-inch chunks
1 medium zucchini, cut
    lengthwise into quarters,
    then crosswise into thirds
1 tablespoon olive oil
6 green onions

4 servings

In small bowl, combine Italian seasoning and salt. Sprinkle both sides of steak evenly with ¼ teaspoon seasoning mixture. Set remaining seasoning mixture aside. Place steak on rack in broiler pan. Set aside.

In 2-quart casserole, combine eggplant, red pepper and zucchini. Add oil to remaining seasoning mixture. Mix well. Drizzle oil mixture over vegetables. Stir to coat. Cover. Microwave at High for 7 to 9 minutes, or until vegetables are tender-crisp, stirring twice. Arrange vegetable mixture and onions evenly around steak. Place steak and vegetables under conventional broiler, with surface of meat 3 to 4 inches from heat. Broil for 15 to 18 minutes, or until vegetables are tender and meat is desired doneness, turning steak over and rearranging vegetables once.

Serving suggestion: Serve with warm popovers.

Per Serving: Calories: 233 • Protein: 26 g • Carbohydrate: 10 g. • Fat: 9 g.
• Cholesterol: 69 mg. • Sodium: 229 mg.
Exchanges: 3 lean meat, 2 vegetable

Broiled Steak & Vegetable Pasta Toss

8 oz. uncooked mostaccioli

2 medium zucchini squash, cut lengthwise into quarters, then crosswise into 1½-inch lengths

1 medium yellow summer squash, cut lengthwise into quarters, then crosswise into 1½-inch lengths

1 small red onion, cut into 8 wedges

1 medium tomato, cut into 8 wedges

2 tablespoons olive oil, divided

2 tablespoons snipped fresh oregano or basil leaves, divided

1- lb. well-trimmed beef top round steak, 1 inch thick

4 servings

Serving suggestion: Serve with hearty whole-grain rolls.

Per Serving: Calories: 480 • Protein: 37 g. • Carbohydrate: 55 g. • Fat: 12 g. • Cholesterol: 71 mg. • Sodium: 65 mg. Exchanges: 2¾ starch, 3 lean meat, 2¾ vegetable, ½ fat

How to Make Broiled Steak & Vegetable Pasta Toss

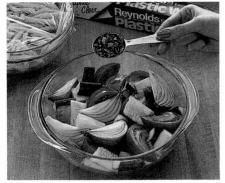

Prepare mostaccioli as directed on package. Rinse and drain. Place in large mixing bowl or salad bowl. Set aside. In 2-quart casserole, combine squashes, onion, tomato, 1 tablespoon oil and 1 tablespoon oregano. Toss to coat. Cover. Microwave at High for 6 to 9 minutes, or until vegetables are tender-crisp, stirring once or twice.

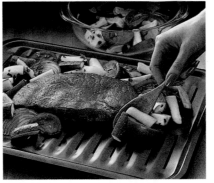

Place steak on rack in broiler pan. Arrange vegetables evenly around steak. Place under conventional broiler, with surface of meat 3 to 4 inches from heat. Broil for 13 to 15 minutes, or until meat is desired doneness, turning meat over and rearranging vegetables once.

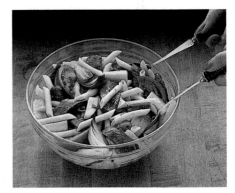

Carve steak across grain into 2 × ¼-inch strips. Add meat and vegetables to mostaccioli. Add remaining 1 tablespoon oil and oregano to mostaccioli. Toss to combine.

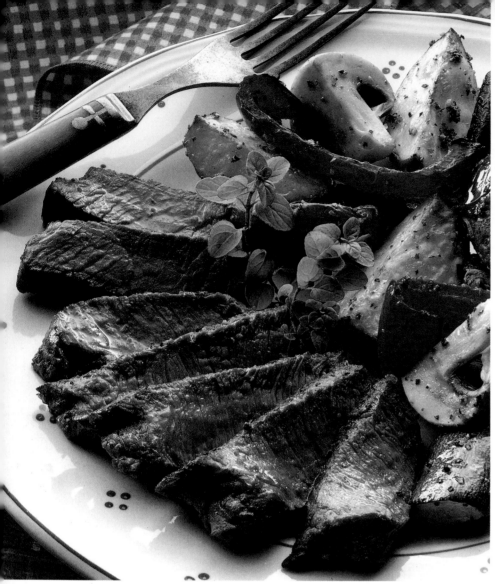

◄ ## Steak & Vegetable Dinner

- 10 small new potatoes, cut into quarters (about 1 lb.)
- ¼ cup water
- 4 large fresh mushrooms, quartered
- 2 medium zucchini, cut lengthwise into thirds, then crosswise into 1½-inch lengths
- 1 medium red pepper, cut lengthwise into eighths
- 2 tablespoons olive oil
- 1 tablespoon plus 1 teaspoon salt-free herb seasoning, divided
- 1- lb. well-trimmed beef top sirloin steak, 1 inch thick

4 servings

In 2-quart casserole, combine potatoes and water. Cover. Microwave at High for 6 to 8 minutes, or until potatoes are tender-crisp. Drain. In large mixing bowl, combine potatoes, mushrooms, zucchini, red pepper, oil and 1 tablespoon herb seasoning. Toss to combine. Set aside.

Sprinkle both sides of steak evenly with remaining 1 teaspoon herb seasoning. Place steak on rack in broiler pan. Arrange vegetables evenly around steak.

Place under conventional broiler, with surface of meat 3 to 4 inches from heat. Broil for 15 to 18 minutes, or until vegetables are tender and meat is desired doneness, turning steak over and rearranging vegetables once.

Serving suggestion: Serve with brown-and-serve dinner rolls or soft bread sticks.

Per Serving: Calories: 358 • Protein: 30 g.
• Carbohydrate: 29 g. • Fat: 14 g.
• Cholesterol: 76 mg. • Sodium: 74 mg.
Exchanges: 1¼ starch, 3 lean meat,
2 vegetable, 1 fat

Broiled Eye Round Dinner

- 2 medium onions, each cut into 8 wedges
- ¼ cup water
- 4 beef eye round steaks (4 oz. each), ¾ inch thick
- 1 medium green pepper, cut into 1-inch chunks
- 1 medium tomato, sliced
- ½ cup low-fat French dressing
- 2 tablespoons red wine

4 servings

In 2-quart casserole, combine onions and water. Cover. Microwave at High for 4 to 5 minutes, or until onions are tender-crisp, stirring once. Drain. Place steaks on rack in broiler pan. Arrange onions, green pepper and tomato evenly around steaks. In 1-cup measure, combine dressing and wine. Brush steaks and vegetables evenly with half of dressing mixture. Place under conventional broiler, with surface of meat 3 to 4 inches from heat. Broil for 13 to 15 minutes, or until meat is desired doneness, turning steaks over, rearranging vegetables and brushing steaks and vegetables once with remaining dressing mixture.

Serving suggestion: Serve with Caesar salad.

Per Serving: Calories: 222 • Protein: 26 g. • Carbohydrate: 11 g. • Fat: 8 g.
• Cholesterol: 59 mg. • Sodium: 357 mg.
Exchanges: 3 lean meat, 1 vegetable, ½ fruit

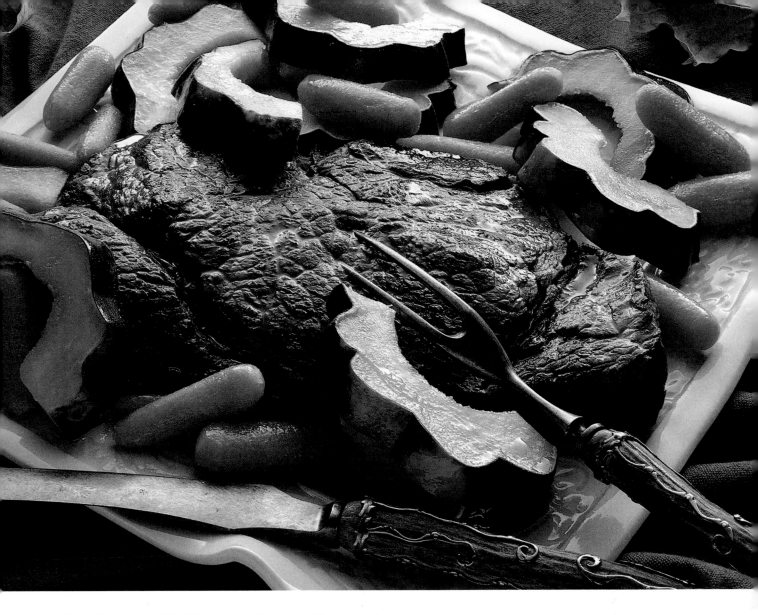

Broiled Sirloin with Harvest Roasted Vegetables

2 tablespoons margarine or
    butter
2 teaspoons packed brown
    sugar
1 acorn squash (1½ lbs.)
2 tablespoons water
1 pkg. (9 oz.) frozen whole
    baby carrots
1- lb. well-trimmed beef top
    sirloin steak, 1 inch thick

4 servings

In small bowl, microwave margarine at High for 45 seconds to 1 minute, or until melted. Add sugar. Mix well. Set aside. Pierce squash twice with fork. Place in microwave oven. Microwave at High for 5 to 6 minutes, or just until squash is warm. (This makes it easier to slice squash.) Slice squash crosswise into ½-inch slices. Cut each slice in half. Remove and discard seeds and pulp.

Place squash in 10-inch square casserole. Add water. Cover. Microwave at High for 5 minutes. Rearrange squash and add carrots. Re-cover. Microwave at High for 5 to 7 minutes, or until squash is tender, stirring once. Place steak on rack in broiler pan. Place under conventional broiler, with surface of meat 3 to 4 inches from heat. Broil for 7 minutes. Turn steak over. Arrange squash and carrots evenly around steak. Brush vegetables evenly with sugar mixture. Broil for 8 to 11 minutes, or until meat is desired doneness and vegetables are lightly browned.

Serving suggestion: Serve with tossed green salad or steamed fresh spinach leaves.

Per Serving: Calories: 302 • Protein: 28 g. • Carbohydrate: 21 g. • Fat: 12 g.
• Cholesterol: 76 mg. • Sodium: 165 mg.
Exchanges: 1 starch, 3 lean meat, 1 vegetable, ½ fat

Teriyaki Steak & Vegetable Kabobs ▶

1 - lb. well-trimmed beef top round steak, 1 inch thick
1 small green pepper, cut into 8 chunks (1-inch chunks)
8 pearl onions, peeled
4 small new potatoes, halved (about 6 oz.)
16 cherry tomatoes

⅓ cup reduced-sodium teriyaki sauce
2 tablespoons packed brown sugar
½ teaspoon ground ginger

4 servings

Serving suggestion: Serve on bed of hot cooked rice.

Per Serving: Calories: 256 • Protein: 30 g. • Carbohydrate: 23 g. • Fat: 4 g. • Cholesterol: 71 mg. • Sodium: 457 mg. Exchanges: ½ starch, 3 lean meat, 2 vegetable, ¼ fruit

How to Make Teriyaki Steak & Vegetable Kabobs

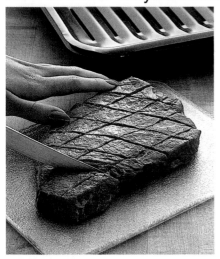

Soak eight 6-inch wooden skewers in water for ½ hour. Score top of steak in diamond pattern, cutting ⅛ inch deep. Place steak scored-side-up on rack in broiler pan. Set aside.

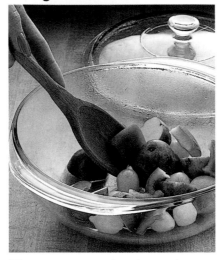

Place pepper chunks, onions and potatoes in 2-quart casserole. Cover. Microwave at High for 6 to 8 minutes, or until potatoes are tender, stirring once.

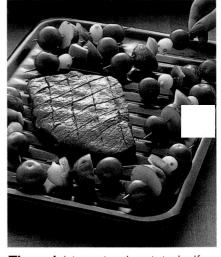

Thread 1 tomato, 1 potato half, 1 pepper chunk, 1 onion and 1 tomato on each skewer. Arrange kabobs evenly around steak on broiler pan. Set aside.

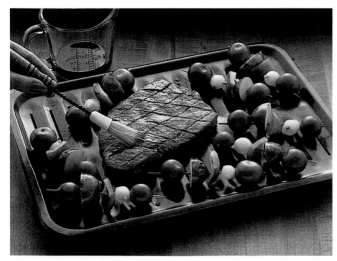

Combine teriyaki sauce, sugar and ginger in 2-cup measure. Microwave at High for 2 to 3 minutes, or until sugar is dissolved, stirring once. Brush steak and kabobs with half of teriyaki mixture.

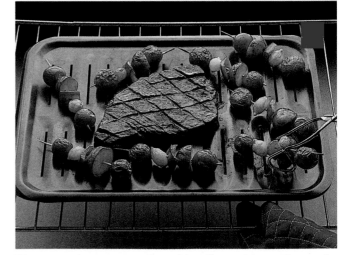

Place under conventional broiler, with surface of meat 3 to 4 inches from heat. Broil for 14 to 16 minutes, or until meat is desired doneness, turning kabobs over and brushing steak and kabobs once with remaining teriyaki mixture.

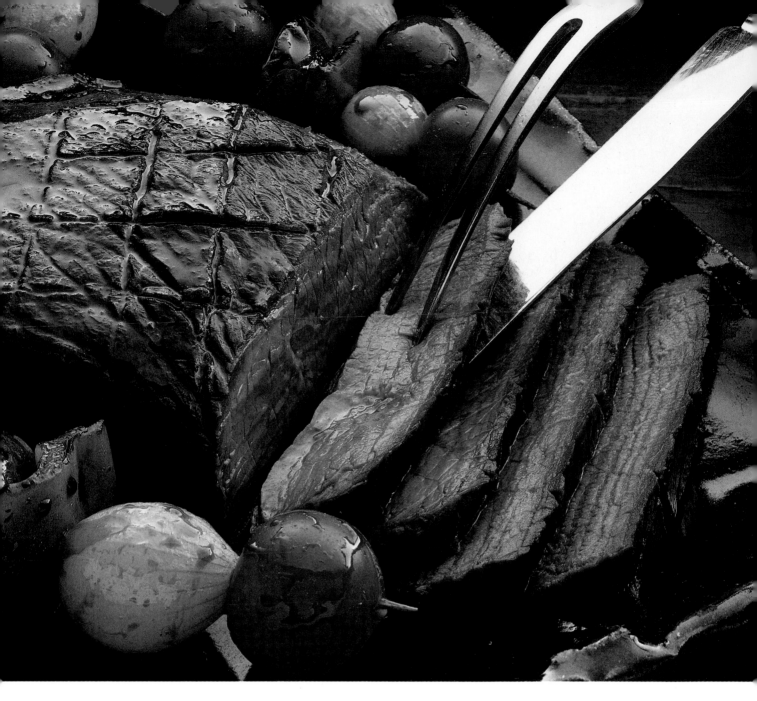

Peppered Beef Steaks with Mushroom & Mustard Sauce

4 oz. fresh mushrooms, sliced
   (1 cup)
2 teaspoons coarsely ground
   fresh black pepper
4 beef eye round steaks
   (4 oz. each), ¾ inch thick
¼ cup sliced green onions
¼ cup white wine
½ cup milk
1 tablespoon Dijon mustard

4 servings

Place mushrooms in 1-quart casserole. Cover. Microwave at High for 5 to 6 minutes, or until tender, stirring once. Drain. Set aside. Sprinkle pepper on sheet of wax paper or microwave cooking paper. Roll edge of each steak evenly in pepper to coat. Spray 10-inch nonstick skillet with nonstick vegetable cooking spray. Heat skillet conventionally over medium-high heat. Cook steaks for 4 to 5 minutes, or until desired doneness, turning over once. Remove steaks from skillet. Cover to keep warm. Set aside. Reduce heat to medium. Add mushrooms, onions and wine to skillet. Stir in milk and mustard. Cook over medium heat for 1 to 3 minutes, or until sauce is reduced by half, stirring constantly. Serve steaks with mushroom sauce.

Serving suggestion: Serve steaks on lightly buttered toast points.

Per Serving: Calories: 186 • Protein: 26 g. • Carbohydrate: 4 g. • Fat: 7 g.
• Cholesterol: 66 mg. • Sodium: 190 mg.
Exchanges: 3 lean meat, ½ vegetable

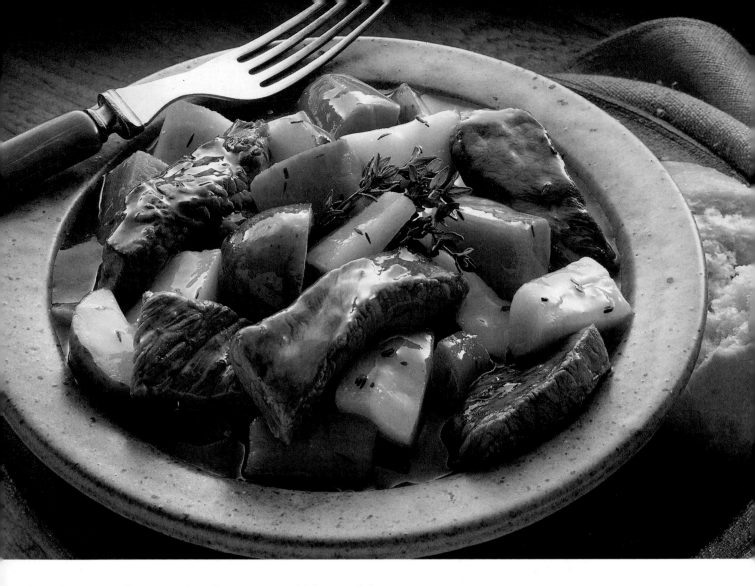

Speedy Sirloin with Pot-roasted Vegetables

5 small new potatoes, cut into 1-inch cubes (about 8 oz.)
2 medium parsnips, cut in half lengthwise, then crosswise into 1-inch lengths
1 medium carrot, cut lengthwise into quarters, then crosswise into 1-inch lengths
1 can (10½ oz.) condensed beef broth, divided
1 - lb. well-trimmed beef top sirloin steak, 1 inch thick, cut into 2 × ¼-inch-thick strips
1 tablespoon cornstarch
½ teaspoon dried thyme leaves
¼ cup dry red wine

4 servings

In 2-quart casserole, combine potatoes, parsnips, carrot and ¼ cup broth. Cover. Microwave at High for 9 to 11 minutes, or until potatoes are tender, stirring twice. Set aside.

Spray 10-inch nonstick skillet with nonstick vegetable cooking spray. Heat skillet conventionally over medium-high heat. Add beef strips. Cook for 5 to 7 minutes, or just until meat is only slightly pink, stirring frequently. Add meat to vegetables in casserole. Cover to keep warm. Set aside.

In 2-cup measure, combine cornstarch and thyme. Blend in remaining broth and the wine. Pour mixture into same skillet. Cook over medium-high heat for 2 to 4 minutes, or until mixture is thickened and translucent and slightly reduced, stirring constantly. Add meat mixture to sauce. Stir to coat.

Serving suggestion: Serve with crusty French bread or hot cooked saffron or white rice.

Per Serving: Calories: 270 • Protein: 28 g. • Carbohydrate: 24 g. • Fat: 6 g.
• Cholesterol: 69 mg. • Sodium: 621 mg.
Exchanges: 1 starch, 3 lean meat, 1 vegetable, ¼ fruit

Quick Beef Goulash ▶

1 - lb. well-trimmed beef top round steak, ½ to ¾ inch thick, cut across grain into 1½ × ¼-inch-thick strips
1 can (16 oz.) stewed tomatoes
1 medium onion, thinly sliced (1 cup)
1 medium green pepper, cut into ¼-inch strips (1 cup)
1 can (6 oz.) tomato paste
1 tablespoon paprika
1 teaspoon caraway seed
¼ teaspoon salt

4 servings

In 3-quart casserole, microwave beef strips at High for 5 to 7 minutes, or just until meat is only slightly pink, stirring twice. Drain. Remove meat from casserole. Set aside. In same casserole, combine remaining ingredients. Cover. Microwave at High for 10 to 13 minutes, or until vegetables are tender and mixture is hot, stirring once. Add meat. Mix well. Cover. Microwave at High for 1 to 2 minutes, or until hot.

Serving suggestion: Serve over hot cooked egg noodles.

Per Serving: Calories: 249 • Protein: 31 g. • Carbohydrate: 22 g. • Fat: 5 g. • Cholesterol: 71 mg. • Sodium: 814 mg. Exchanges: 3 lean meat, 3 vegetable

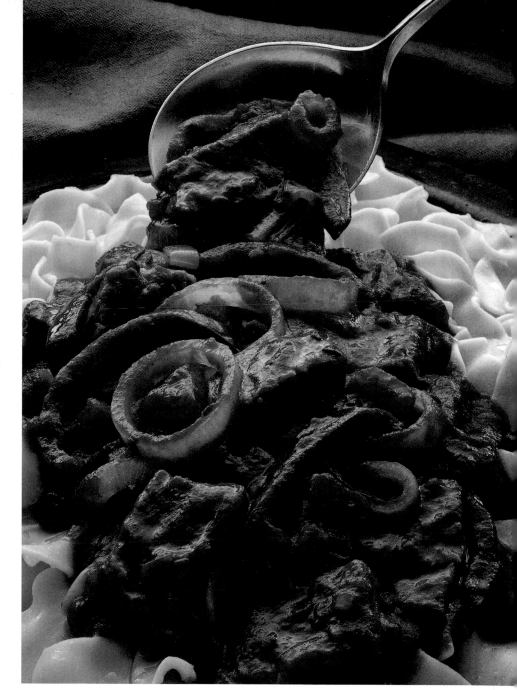

Steak & Mushroom Pizza

4 pita loaves (7-inch)
2 cups shredded mozzarella cheese
¼ cup snipped fresh basil leaves
1 to 2 cloves garlic, minced
1 - lb. well-trimmed beef top sirloin steak, 1 inch thick, cut into 2 × ¼-inch-thick strips
8 oz. fresh mushrooms, sliced (2 cups)
¾ cup thinly sliced red or green pepper strips

4 servings

Heat conventional oven to 425°F. Arrange pitas on large baking sheets. In medium mixing bowl, combine cheese, basil and garlic. Sprinkle cheese mixture evenly over pitas. Set aside. In 2-quart casserole, combine beef strips and mushrooms. Microwave at High for 6 to 8 minutes, or just until meat is only slightly pink, stirring twice. Drain. Spoon meat mixture evenly over pitas. Top evenly with pepper strips. Bake conventionally for 10 to 12 minutes, or until cheese is melted and pizzas are hot.

Serving suggestion: Serve with sliced fresh tomatoes topped with peppery Italian dressing.

Per Serving: Calories: 522 • Protein: 44 g. • Carbohydrate: 43 g. • Fat: 19 g. • Cholesterol: 120 mg. • Sodium: 634 mg. Exchanges: 2 starch, 5 lean meat, 1 vegetable, 1 fat

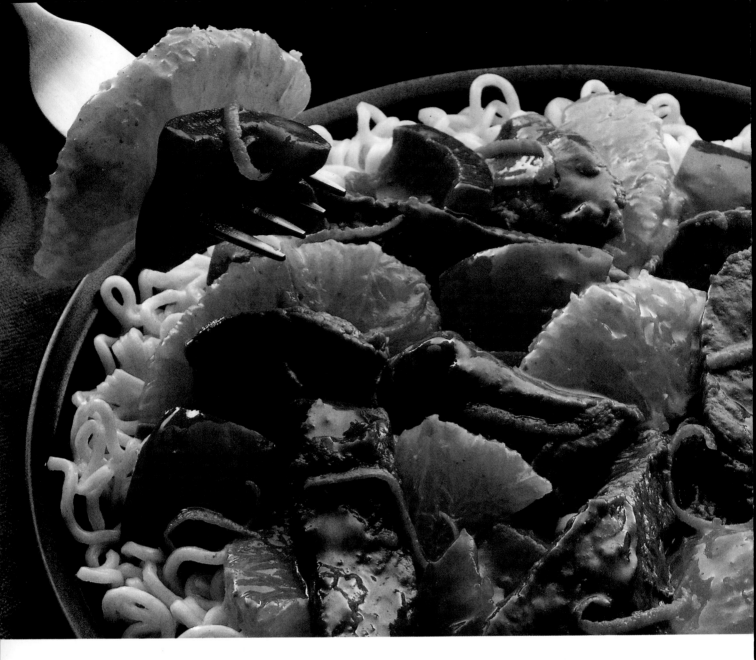

Spicy Beef with Peppers & Oranges

1 - lb. well-trimmed beef top
    sirloin steak, 1 inch thick,
    cut into 2 × 1/8-inch-thick
    strips
1 medium seedless orange
1/2 teaspoon ground ginger
1/4 teaspoon cayenne
1 tablespoon reduced-sodium
    soy sauce
1 teaspoon cornstarch
2 cups red or green pepper
    chunks (3/4-inch chunks)

4 servings

Place beef strips in 3-quart casserole. Set aside. Grate 1 teaspoon peel from orange. Set aside. Remove and discard remaining peel. Slice orange into 1/4-inch slices. Cut each slice in half. Set aside. Sprinkle meat with reserved peel, the ginger, cayenne and soy sauce. Toss to coat. Cover. Microwave at High for 4 to 7 minutes, or just until meat is only slightly pink, stirring once or twice. Using slotted spoon, remove meat from casserole. Set aside.

Add cornstarch to liquid in casserole. Stir until smooth. Add pepper chunks. Re-cover. Microwave at High for 4 to 5 minutes, or until mixture is thickened and translucent and peppers are tender-crisp, stirring once or twice. Stir in meat and orange pieces. Re-cover. Microwave at High for 1 to 2 minutes, or until hot.

Serving suggestion: Serve over hot cooked ramen noodles, fine egg noodles or rice.

Per Serving: Calories: 186 • Protein: 25 g. • Carbohydrate: 9 g. • Fat: 5 g.
• Cholesterol: 69 mg. • Sodium: 217 mg.
Exchanges: 3 lean meat, 1 vegetable, 1/4 fruit

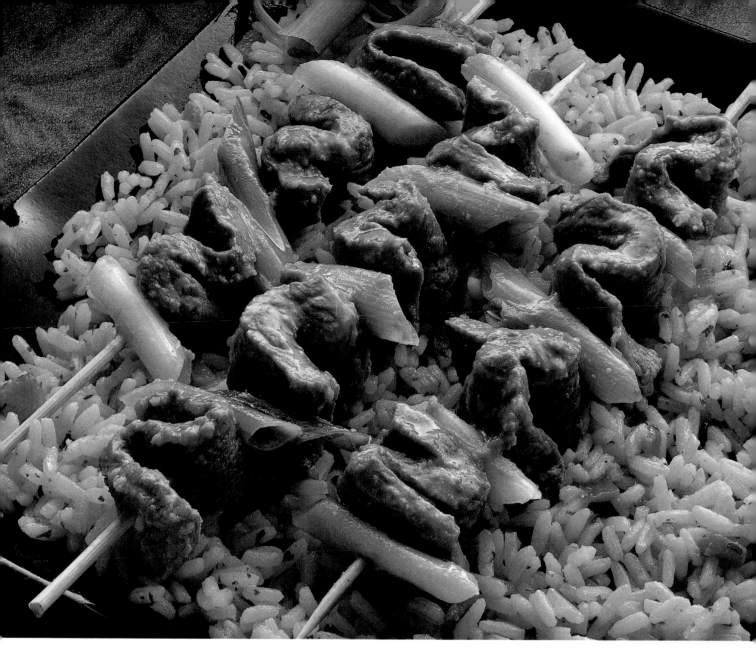

Skewered Beef Satay

¼ cup ready-to-serve chicken
   broth
3 tablespoons fresh lime juice
2 tablespoons creamy
   peanut butter
1 tablespoon reduced-sodium
   soy sauce
2 teaspoons sugar
1 teaspoon Chinese hot
   pepper oil
1 - lb. well-trimmed beef top
   round steak, 1 inch thick,
   cut into 2 × ¼-inch-thick
   strips
4 green onions, cut into 1-inch
   lengths (½ cup)

4 servings

In 2-cup measure, combine broth, juice, peanut butter, soy sauce, sugar and hot pepper oil. Microwave at High for 2 to 2½ minutes, or until mixture is hot and can be stirred smooth, stirring once.

Place beef strips in medium mixing bowl. Add half of peanut butter mixture. Stir to coat. Set remaining peanut butter mixture aside. Let beef mixture stand at room temperature for 5 minutes. Drain.

Thread meat and onions evenly onto twelve 8-inch wooden skewers. Arrange kabobs in even layer on 12-inch plate. Brush with half of remaining peanut butter mixture. Cover with wax paper or microwave cooking paper. Microwave at High for 6 to 8 minutes, or just until meat is only slightly pink, rearranging and basting kabobs with remaining peanut butter mixture once.

Serving suggestion: Serve on bed of seasoned rice.

Per Serving: Calories: 211 • Protein: 29 g. • Carbohydrate: 4 g. • Fat: 8 g.
• Cholesterol: 71 mg. • Sodium: 240 mg.
Exchanges: ¼ starch, 3⅓ lean meat

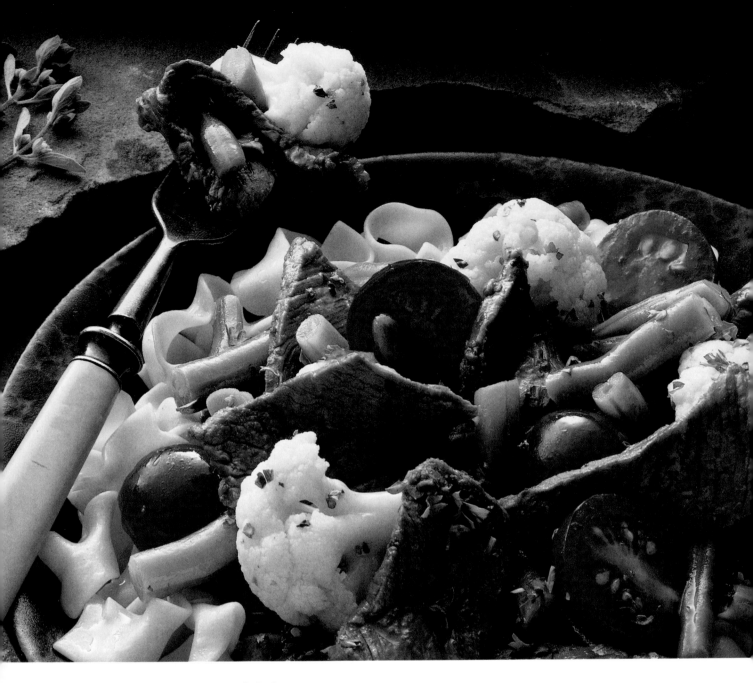

Easy Beef & Vegetable Stir-fry

1 - lb. well-trimmed beef top
    sirloin steak, 1 inch thick,
    cut into 2 × ⅛-inch-thick
    strips
2 cups fresh cauliflowerets
1 cup frozen cut green beans
1 tablespoon olive oil
½ teaspoon dried marjoram
    leaves
¼ teaspoon garlic salt
1 cup halved cherry tomatoes
    Snipped fresh parsley
    (optional)

4 servings

In 3-quart casserole, microwave beef strips at High for 4 to 6 minutes, or just until meat is only slightly pink, stirring once. Drain. Remove meat from casserole. Set aside. In same casserole, place cauliflower, beans, oil, marjoram and garlic salt. Cover. Microwave at High for 5 to 6 minutes, or until vegetables are tender, stirring once. Stir in meat. Microwave at High, uncovered, for 2 to 3 minutes, or until hot. Stir in tomatoes. Sprinkle with parsley.

Serving suggestion: Serve with hot cooked egg noodles.

Per Serving: Calories: 223 • Protein: 28 g. • Carbohydrate: 6 g. • Fat: 10 g.
• Cholesterol: 76 mg. • Sodium: 180 mg.
Exchanges: 3 lean meat, 1 vegetable

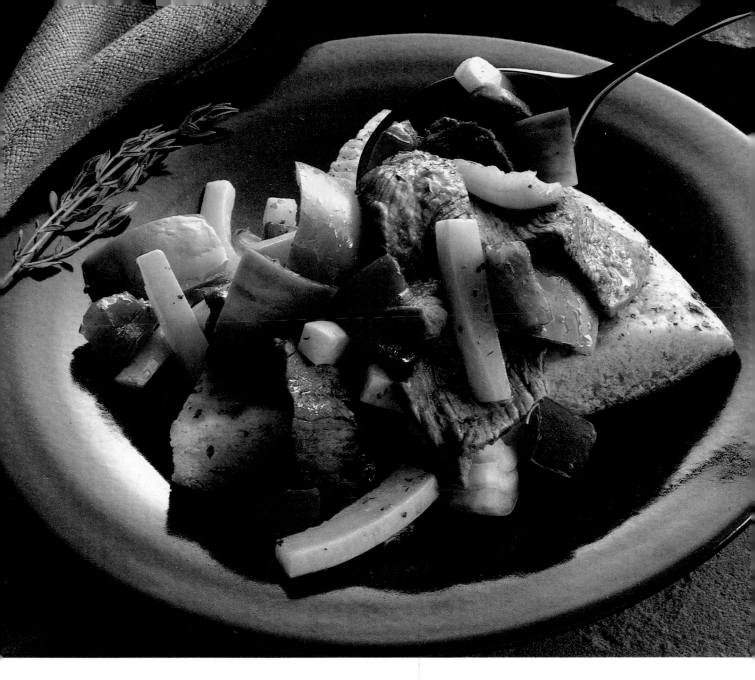

Italian Beef Stir-fry

1 - lb. well-trimmed
    boneless beef sirloin
    steak, 1 inch thick, cut into
    2 × 1/8-inch-thick strips
1/2 cup red onion chunks
    (1-inch chunks)
1 tablespoon olive oil
1 1/2 cups yellow summer squash
    strips (1 1/2 × 1/4-inch strips)
1 cup red or green pepper
    chunks (1-inch chunks)
1/2 teaspoon Italian seasoning
1/8 teaspoon garlic powder
1 cup seeded chopped
    tomato

4 servings

Place beef strips in 3-quart casserole. Cover. Microwave at High for 5 to 6 minutes, or just until meat is only slightly pink, stirring once or twice. Drain. Remove meat from casserole. Set aside.

In same casserole, combine onions and oil. Cover. Microwave at High for 1 to 2 minutes, or until onion is tender-crisp. Stir in remaining ingredients, except meat and tomato. Re-cover. Microwave at High for 3 to 4 minutes, or until vegetables are tender-crisp, stirring once. Add meat and tomato. Stir gently. Microwave at High for 1 to 2 minutes, or until hot.

Serving suggestion: Serve with wedges of bakery Focaccia loaf or polenta.

Per Serving: Calories: 172 • Protein: 19 g. • Carbohydrate: 7 g. • Fat: 7 g.
• Cholesterol: 52 mg. • Sodium: 57 mg.
Exchanges: 3 lean meat, 1 1/2 vegetable

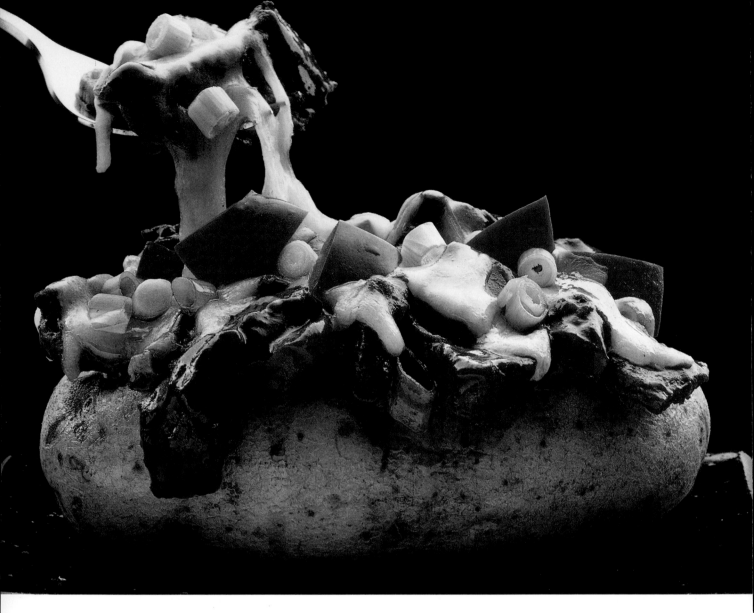

Chunky Beef Barbecue Potato Topper

2   medium baking potatoes
    (8 to 10 oz. each)
1/2 cup plus 2 tablespoons
    sliced green onions,
    divided
1/2 cup plus 2 tablespoons
    chopped red or green
    pepper, divided
1 - lb. well-trimmed beef top
    sirloin steak, 1 inch thick, cut
    into 2 × 1/4-inch-thick strips
3/4 cup barbecue sauce
1/4 cup shredded Monterey
    Jack cheese with jalapeño
    peppers (2 oz.)

4 servings

Pierce potatoes with fork. Arrange on paper towel in microwave oven. Microwave at High for 8 to 13 minutes, or just until tender, rearranging once. Set aside. In 2-quart casserole, combine 1/2 cup onions and 1/2 cup chopped pepper. Cover. Microwave at High for 2 to 3 minutes, or until vegetables are tender-crisp. Stir in beef strips. Microwave at High, uncovered, for 3 to 5 minutes, or just until meat is only slightly pink, stirring once. Drain. Stir in barbecue sauce. Cover. Microwave at High for 4 to 5 minutes, or until hot.

Cut each potato in half lengthwise. Place halves cut-sides-up on individual serving plates. Spoon meat mixture evenly over potato halves. Sprinkle each with 1 tablespoon cheese. Sprinkle evenly with remaining 2 tablespoons onions and chopped pepper. Microwave at High for 30 seconds to 1 minute, or until cheese is melted.

Serving suggestion: Serve with fresh steamed corn on the cob.

Per Serving: Calories: 328 • Protein: 31 g. • Carbohydrate: 27 g. • Fat: 10 g.
• Cholesterol: 84 mg. • Sodium: 550 mg.
Exchanges: 1 starch, 3½ lean meat, 2 vegetable

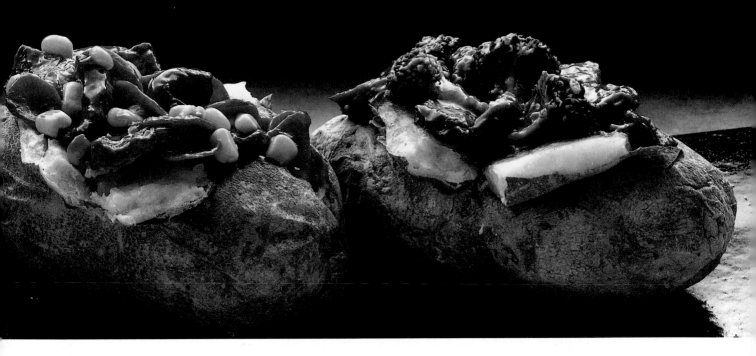

Szechuan-style Beef Potato Topper ▲

4 medium baking potatoes (8 to 10 oz. each)
1- lb. well-trimmed beef top sirloin steak,
   1 inch thick, cut into 2 × ¼-inch-thick strips
2 teaspoons cornstarch
⅛ teaspoon crushed red pepper flakes
⅓ cup reduced-sodium teriyaki sauce
1 cup thinly sliced carrots
½ cup frozen corn

4 servings

Pierce potatoes with fork. Arrange in circle on paper towel in microwave oven. Microwave at High for 10 to 16 minutes, or just until tender, rearranging once. Set aside. In 2-quart casserole, microwave beef strips at High for 5 to 7 minutes, or just until meat is only slightly pink, stirring twice. Using slotted spoon, remove meat from casserole. Set aside.

In small bowl, combine cornstarch and red pepper flakes. Blend in teriyaki sauce. Add to liquid in casserole. Mix well. Add carrots and corn. Mix well. Microwave at High for 4 to 8 minutes, or until mixture is thickened and translucent and carrots are tender, stirring twice. Add meat. Mix well. Microwave at High for 2 to 4 minutes, or until hot, stirring once. Slash each potato lengthwise and then crosswise. Gently press both ends until center pops open. Spoon meat mixture evenly over potatoes.

Serving suggestion: Serve with steamed snow pea pods and red pepper strips.

Per Serving: Calories: 430 • Protein: 31 g. • Carbohydrate: 65 g. • Fat: 5 g. • Cholesterol: 69 mg. • Sodium: 489 mg. Exchanges: 3¼ starch, 3 lean meat, 1 vegetable, ½ fruit

Garlic Beef & Broccoli Potato Topper ▲

4 medium baking potatoes (8 to 10 oz. each)
1- lb. well-trimmed beef top sirloin steak,
   1 inch thick, cut into 2 × ¼-inch-thick strips
2 cloves garlic, minced, divided
1 pkg. (0.87 oz.) brown gravy mix
1 cup cold water
2 cups fresh broccoli flowerets

4 servings

Pierce potatoes with fork. Arrange in circle on paper towel in microwave oven. Microwave at High for 10 to 16 minutes, or just until tender, rearranging once. Set aside. In 2-quart casserole, combine beef strips and half of minced garlic. Microwave at High for 5 to 7 minutes, or just until meat is only slightly pink, stirring twice. Drain. Remove meat from casserole. Set aside.

In same casserole, combine gravy mix and remaining minced garlic. Blend in water. Add broccoli. Mix well. Microwave at High, uncovered, for 7 to 10 minutes, or until mixture is thickened and translucent, stirring 2 or 3 times. Add meat. Mix well. Microwave at High for 2 to 3 minutes, or until hot, stirring once. Slash each potato lengthwise and then crosswise. Gently press both ends until center pops open. Spoon meat mixture evenly over potatoes.

Serving suggestion: Serve with steamed whole baby carrots.

Per Serving: Calories: 437 • Protein: 34 g. • Carbohydrate: 61 g. • Fat: 7 g. • Cholesterol: 76 mg. • Sodium: 390 mg. Exchanges: 3 starch, 3 lean meat, 1 vegetable

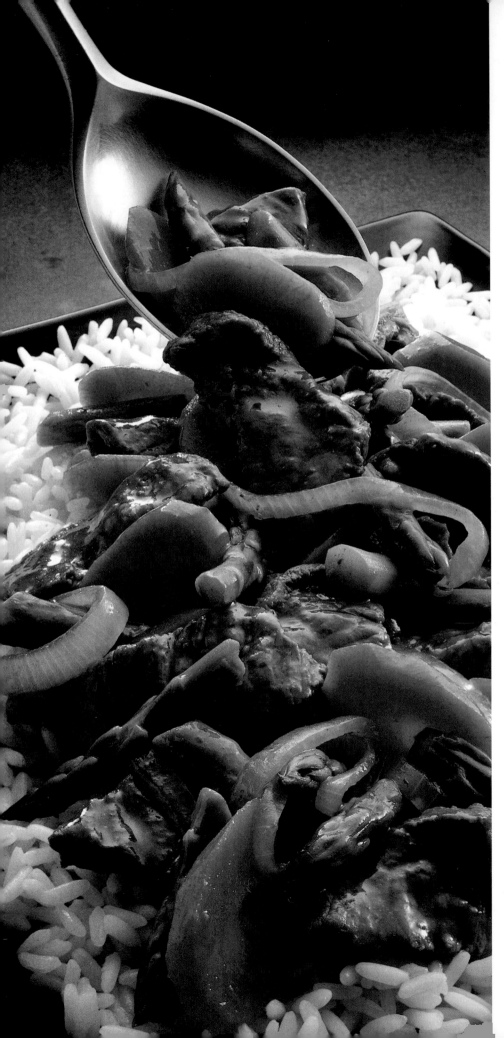

Steak & Asparagus Stir-fry

1-lb. well-trimmed beef top
     round steak, 1 inch thick,
     cut into 2 × ⅛-inch-thick
     strips
1 to 2 teaspoons ground
     ginger
1 teaspoon cornstarch
¼ cup sherry
¼ cup reduced-sodium soy
     sauce
1 lb. fresh asparagus spears,
     cut into 1-inch lengths
1 cup thinly sliced carrots
1 medium onion, sliced and
     separated into rings

4 servings

In 2-quart casserole, microwave
beef strips at High for 5 to 7 minutes, or just until meat is only
slightly pink, stirring twice. Drain.
Remove meat from casserole.
Set aside.

In same casserole, combine
ginger and cornstarch. Blend in
sherry and soy sauce. Add asparagus, carrots and onion. Mix
well. Microwave at High, uncovered, for 8 to 14 minutes, or
until sauce is thickened and
translucent, stirring twice. Add
meat. Mix well. Microwave at High
for 1 to 2 minutes, or until hot.

Serving suggestion: Serve with
hot cooked rice or noodles.

Per Serving: Calories: 222 • Protein: 30 g.
• Carbohydrate: 11 g. • Fat: 4 g.
• Cholesterol: 71 mg. • Sodium: 665 mg.
Exchanges: 3 lean meat, 2 vegetable

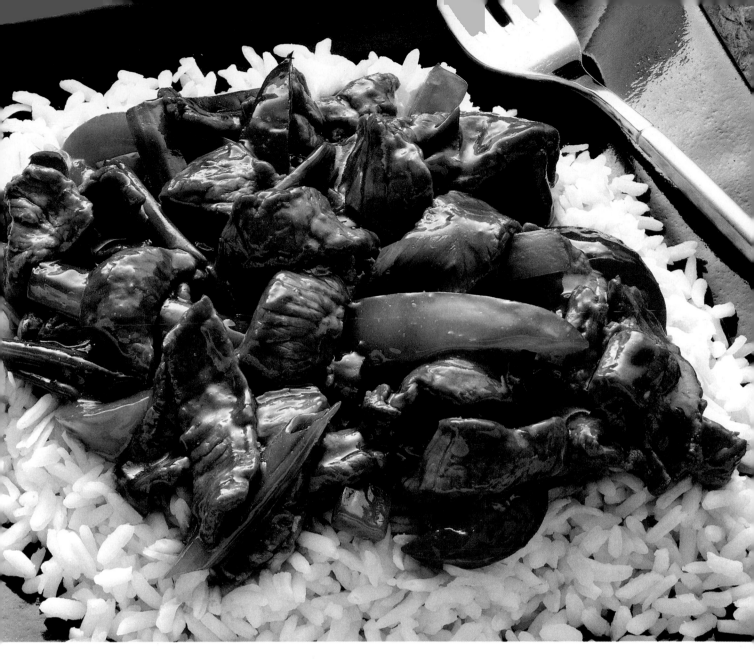

Mongolian Beef & Vegetables

1 - lb. well-trimmed beef
    top round steak, 1/2 to 3/4
    inch thick, cut across grain
    into 2 × 1/8-inch-thick strips
1 tablespoon cornstarch
1 teaspoon sugar
1/3 cup reduced-sodium soy
    sauce
2 tablespoons sherry
3 stalks celery, cut into thin
    strips (3 × 1/4-inch strips)
1 cup thinly sliced red and
    yellow pepper strips
6 green onions, sliced
    diagonally into 1-inch
    lengths (3/4 cup)

4 servings

Place beef strips in 3-quart casserole. Set aside. In small mixing bowl, combine cornstarch and sugar. Blend in soy sauce and sherry. Add soy mixture to meat. Stir to coat. Let stand for 10 minutes. Microwave at High for 4 to 6 minutes, or just until meat is only slightly pink. Using slotted spoon, remove meat from casserole. Set aside. Add vegetables to liquid in casserole. Stir to coat. Microwave at High for 6 to 8 minutes, or until vegetables are tender, stirring 2 or 3 times. Add meat. Mix well. Microwave at High for 2 to 3 minutes, or until hot.

Serving suggestion: Serve with hot cooked rice or noodles.

Per Serving: Calories: 191 • Protein: 28 g. • Carbohydrate: 10 g. • Fat: 4 g.
• Cholesterol: 65 mg. • Sodium: 880 mg.
Exchanges: 3 lean meat, 1 vegetable, 1/3 fruit

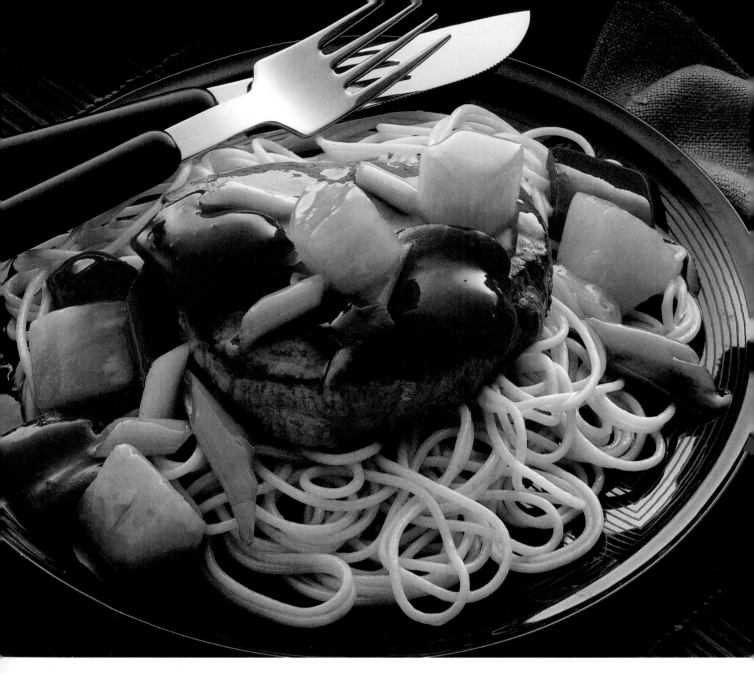

Pineapple Teriyaki Eye Round Steaks

1 cup red or green pepper
   chunks (1-inch chunks)
½ cup sliced green onions
   (½-inch lengths)
½ teaspoon ground ginger,
   divided
2 teaspoons cornstarch
2 tablespoons reduced-
   sodium soy sauce
2 teaspoons honey
1 can (8 oz.) pineapple
   chunks in juice, drained
   (reserve ½ cup juice)
4 beef eye round steaks
   (4 oz. each), ¾ inch thick

4 servings

In 4-cup measure, combine pepper chunks, onions, ¼ teaspoon ginger, the cornstarch, soy sauce, honey and reserved pineapple juice. Microwave at High for 4 to 6 minutes, or until mixture is thickened and translucent, stirring once. Stir in pineapple. Cover with plastic wrap. Set aside. Pound steaks to ½-inch thickness. Sprinkle both sides of steaks evenly with remaining ¼ teaspoon ginger. Spray 10-inch nonstick skillet with nonstick vegetable cooking spray. Heat skillet conventionally over medium-high heat. Cook steaks for 4 to 5 minutes, or until desired doneness, turning over once. Spoon sauce over steaks.

Serving suggestion: Serve with hot cooked vermicelli or fine egg noodles.

Per Serving: Calories: 209 • Protein: 26 g. • Carbohydrate: 16 g. • Fat: 5 g. • Cholesterol: 59 mg. • Sodium: 355 mg.
Exchanges: 3 lean meat, 1 vegetable, ¾ fruit

42

Pineapple Beef

1 - lb. well-trimmed beef
    top sirloin steak, 1 inch
    thick, cut into 2 × 1/4-inch-
    thick strips
1 can (20 oz.) pineapple
    chunks in heavy syrup,
    drained (reserve 1/2 cup
    syrup)
1/4 cup tomato sauce
2 tablespoons cider vinegar
1 tablespoon reduced-sodium
    soy sauce
2 teaspoons cornstarch
6 oz. fresh snow pea pods
    (2 cups)
1 cup red pepper chunks
    (1-inch chunks)

4 servings

In 2-quart casserole, microwave beef strips at High for 5 to 7 minutes, or just until meat is only slightly pink, stirring twice. Drain. Remove meat from casserole. Set aside.

In same casserole, combine reserved pineapple syrup, the tomato sauce, vinegar, soy sauce and cornstarch. Add pea pods and pepper chunks. Mix well. Microwave at High for 6 to 8 minutes, or until sauce is thickened and translucent, stirring once or twice. Add meat and pineapple chunks to sauce mixture. Mix well. Microwave at High for 2 to 3 minutes, or until hot, stirring once.

Serving suggestion: Serve over hot cooked rice.

Per Serving: Calories: 314 • Protein: 28 g. • Carbohydrate: 36 g. • Fat: 6 g. • Cholesterol: 76 mg. • Sodium: 302 mg. Exchanges: 3 lean meat, 1 vegetable, 2 fruit

Beef & Barley Stuffed Peppers*▲

1 cup uncooked quick
    pearled barley
4 medium green peppers
1/4 cup water
1 - lb. well-trimmed beef
    top round steak, 1/2 to
    3/4 inch thick, cut across
    grain into 1 1/2 × 1/4-inch-thick
    strips

1/2 cup chopped onion
1/4 to 1/2 teaspoon dried thyme
    leaves
1 can (15 oz.) tomato sauce
1 can (14 1/2 oz.) diced
    tomatoes, drained

4 servings

Prepare barley as directed on package. Drain. Set aside. Cut 1/4-inch slice from top of each pepper. Remove seeds and membrane. Remove thin slice from bottom of each pepper to allow peppers to stand upright. Arrange peppers cut-sides-up in 8-inch square baking dish. Sprinkle with water. Cover with plastic wrap. Microwave at High for 6 to 8 minutes, or until peppers are tender-crisp, rearranging once. Drain. Set aside.

In 2-quart casserole, combine beef strips, onion and thyme. Microwave at High for 5 to 7 minutes, or just until meat is only slightly pink, stirring once. Drain. Add barley, tomato sauce and tomatoes. Mix well. Spoon barley mixture into peppers. Spoon any remaining mixture around peppers. Re-cover. Microwave at 70% (Medium High) for 13 to 15 minutes, or until hot, rotating dish twice.

Serving suggestion: Serve with mixed green salad.

*Recipe not recommended for ovens with less than 600 cooking watts.

Per Serving: Calories: 360 • Protein: 34 g. • Carbohydrate: 45 g. • Fat: 5 g. • Cholesterol: 71 mg. • Sodium: 865 mg. Exchanges: 2 starch, 3 lean meat, 3 vegetable

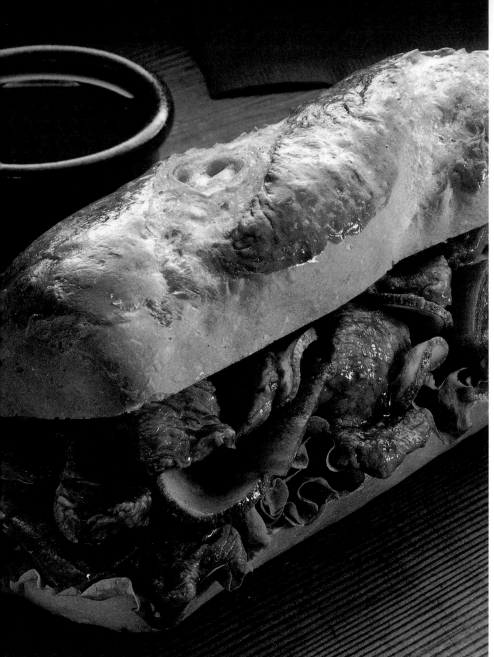

◄ Beef & Vegetable au Jus

    1 cup thinly sliced zucchini
    ½ cup red onion chunks
         (1-inch chunks)
    ¼ cup ready-to-serve beef broth
    2 tablespoons chili sauce
    1- lb. well-trimmed beef
         top sirloin steak, ½ to ¾
         inch thick, cut into
         2 × ⅛-inch-thick strips

4 servings

In 2-quart casserole, combine
zucchini and onion. Cover. Microwave at High for 3 to 4 minutes,
or until vegetables are tender-
crisp. Set aside. In 1-cup measure, combine broth and chili
sauce. Add beef strips and broth
mixture to vegetables in casserole. Microwave at High for 4 to
5 minutes, or just until meat is
only slightly pink, stirring once.

Serving suggestions: Spoon meat
mixture and broth over lettuce-
lined hard rolls or over hot baked
potatoes. Serve additional broth
on the side for dipping, if desired.

Per Serving: Calories: 169 • Protein: 25 g.
• Carbohydrate: 5 g. • Fat: 5 g.
• Cholesterol: 69 mg. • Sodium: 233 mg.
Exchanges: 3 lean meat, 1 vegetable

Easy Chunky Spaghetti Sauce

    1- lb. well-trimmed beef
         top round steak, ½ to ¾
         inch thick, cut across grain
         into 1½ × ¼-inch-thick strips
    1 can (14½ oz.) whole
         tomatoes, undrained and
         cut up
    4 oz. fresh mushrooms, sliced
         (1 cup)
    1 can (6 oz.) tomato paste
    ½ cup chopped green pepper
    1 teaspoon Italian seasoning
    1 teaspoon sugar
    ¼ teaspoon garlic powder

4 servings

Place beef strips in 3-quart casserole. Microwave at High for 5 to 7
minutes, or just until meat is only slightly pink, stirring twice. Drain.
Remove meat from casserole. Set aside. In same casserole, combine
remaining ingredients. Cover. Microwave at High for 10 to 13 minutes, or until green pepper is tender, stirring once or twice. Add meat.
Mix well. Re-cover. Microwave at High for 1 to 2 minutes, or until hot.

Serving suggestion: Serve over hot cooked spaghetti.

Per Serving: Calories: 223 • Protein: 30 g. • Carbohydrate: 15 g. • Fat: 5 g.
• Cholesterol: 71 mg. • Sodium: 561 mg.
Exchanges: 3 lean meat, 3 vegetable

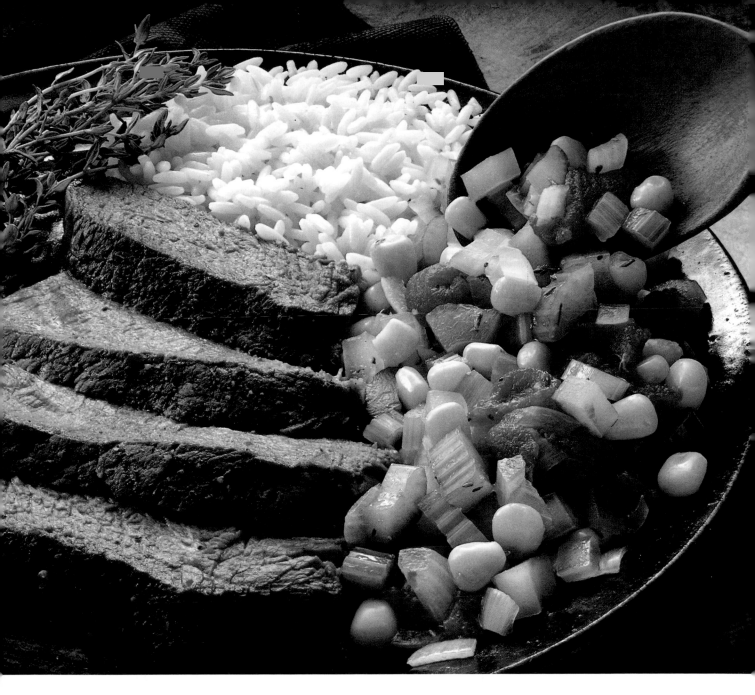

Sirloin with Creole Salsa

1 can (8 oz.) whole tomatoes,
   undrained and chopped
½ cup sliced celery
½ cup chopped onion
½ cup frozen corn
¼ teaspoon dried thyme
   leaves
8 drops red pepper sauce
1- lb. well-trimmed beef
   top sirloin steak, 1 inch thick
½ teaspoon seasoned pepper
   medley, divided

4 servings

In 4-cup measure, combine all ingredients, except steak and ¼ teaspoon seasoned pepper medley. Microwave at High for 6 to 8 minutes, or until vegetables are tender-crisp, stirring once or twice. Cover with plastic wrap. Set salsa aside. Sprinkle both sides of steak evenly with remaining ¼ teaspoon seasoned pepper medley. Place steak on rack in broiler pan. Place under conventional broiler, with surface of meat 3 to 4 inches from heat. Broil for 15 to 18 minutes, or until desired doneness, turning over once. Carve steak into thin slices. Serve with salsa.

Serving suggestion: Serve with hot cooked rice or baked potatoes.

Per Serving: Calories: 206 • Protein: 27 g. • Carbohydrate: 9 g. • Fat: 6 g.
• Cholesterol: 76 mg. • Sodium: 169 mg.
Exchanges: ⅓ starch, 3 lean meat, 1 vegetable

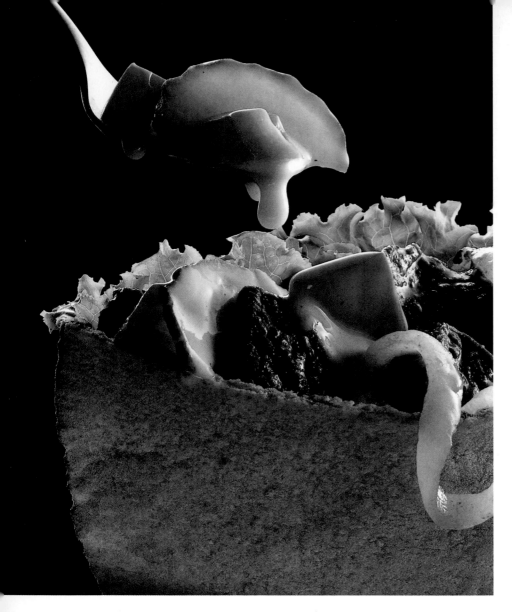

Greek Steak & Pita Sandwiches ▲

½ cup low-fat creamy
   cucumber dressing
½ medium cucumber, cut
   lengthwise in half and sliced
½ cup seeded chopped
   tomato
1- lb. well-trimmed beef top
   sirloin steak, 1 inch thick,
   cut into 2 × ¼-inch-thick
   strips

1 small onion, sliced and
   separated into rings
1 clove garlic, minced
½ teaspoon dried oregano
   leaves
4 pita loaves (6-inch), split

4 servings

In small mixing bowl, combine dressing, cucumber and tomato. Set
aside. In 2-quart casserole, combine beef strips, onion, garlic and
oregano. Microwave at High for 6 to 8 minutes, or just until meat is
only slightly pink, stirring once. Drain. Line pitas with leaf lettuce, if
desired. Spoon meat mixture and cucumber mixture evenly into pitas.

Serving suggestion: Serve with carrot sticks and Greek olives.

Per Serving: Calories: 413 • Protein: 32 g. • Carbohydrate: 42 g. • Fat: 13 g.
• Cholesterol: 76 mg. • Sodium: 842 mg.
Exchanges: 2½ starch, 3 lean meat, 1 vegetable, 1 fat

Fajita Pitas

1- lb. well-trimmed boneless
   beef sirloin steak, ¾ inch
   thick, cut into 2 × ⅛-inch-
   thick strips
¼ cup reduced-sodium
   teriyaki sauce
1 tablespoon fresh lime juice
1 tablespoon canned diced
   jalapeño peppers (optional)
2 cups thinly sliced red and
   green pepper strips
1 cup sliced red onion
1 teaspoon olive oil
4 pita loaves (6-inch), split

4 servings

Place beef strips in medium mixing bowl. Add teriyaki sauce,
juice and jalapeño peppers. Mix
well. Marinate at room temperature for 10 minutes.

In 2-quart casserole, combine
pepper strips, onion and oil. Microwave at High, uncovered, for 3
to 5 minutes, or until vegetables
are tender-crisp, stirring once.
Add meat mixture. Mix well.
Microwave at High, uncovered,
for 5 to 7 minutes, or just until
meat is only slightly pink, stirring
twice. Line pitas with fresh
spinach leaves, if desired. Spoon
meat mixture evenly into pitas.

Serving suggestion: Serve with
hot and spicy refried beans.

Per Serving: Calories: 374 • Protein: 31 g.
• Carbohydrate: 45 g. • Fat: 7 g.
• Cholesterol: 69 mg. • Sodium: 731 mg.
Exchanges: 2¼ starch, 3 lean meat,
1½ vegetable, ¼ fruit

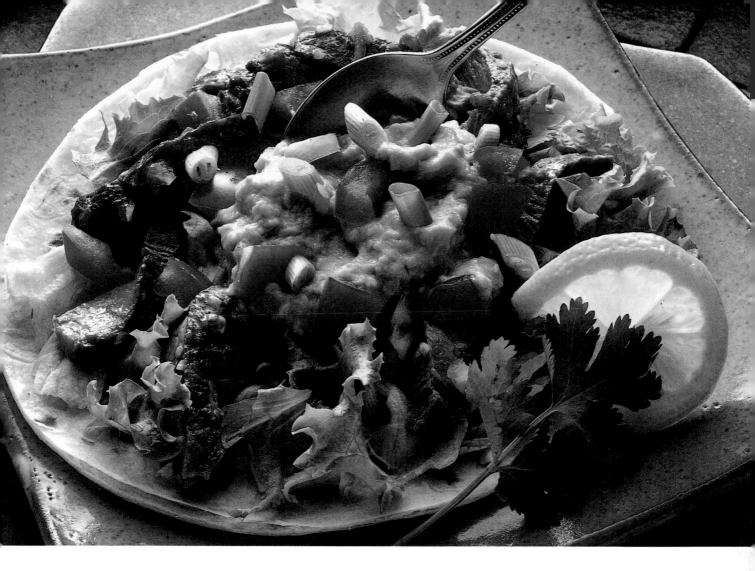

Beef Tostada ▲

4 flour tortillas (8-inch)
1- lb. well-trimmed beef top
   sirloin steak, 1 inch thick,
   cut into 2 × ¼-inch-thick
   strips
1 clove garlic, minced

1 teaspoon ground cumin
1½ cups salsa
4 cups shredded lettuce
   Low-calorie Guacamole
   (right), optional

4 servings

Place 2 tortillas on baking sheet. Place under conventional broiler, with surface of tortillas 5 to 6 inches from heat. Broil for 2 to 4 minutes, or until lightly browned, turning over once. Repeat with remaining tortillas. Set aside. In 2-quart casserole, combine beef strips, garlic and cumin. Microwave at High for 5 to 7 minutes, or just until meat is only slightly pink, stirring once. Drain. Add salsa to meat in casserole. Mix well. Place 1 cup lettuce on each tortilla. Top each with one-fourth of meat mixture and 3 tablespoons guacamole. Sprinkle with seeded chopped tomato and sliced green onions, if desired.

Serving suggestion: Serve with melon slices sprinkled with fresh lime juice.

Per Serving: Calories: 368 • Protein: 32 g. • Carbohydrate: 36 g. • Fat: 10 g.
• Cholesterol: 76 mg. • Sodium: 948 mg.
Exchanges: 1½ starch, 3 lean meat, 2½ vegetable, ⅔ fat

Low-calorie Guacamole ▲

½ medium avocado (about
   3 oz.)
½ cup plain nonfat yogurt
1 teaspoon lemon juice
¼ teaspoon garlic salt
⅛ teaspoon cayenne

4 servings

In small mixing bowl, mash avocado with fork until smooth. Add remaining ingredients. Mix well. Serve guacamole with Beef Tostada, left.

Per Serving: Calories: 51 • Protein: 2 g.
• Carbohydrate: 4 g. • Fat: 3 g.
• Cholesterol: 1 mg. • Sodium: 137 mg.
Exchanges: ⅔ fat

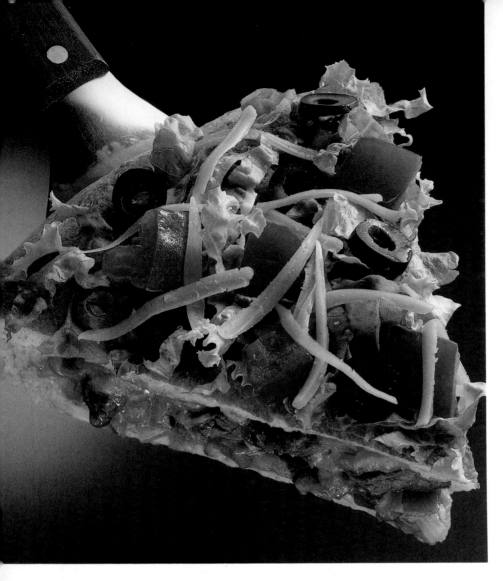

Stuffed Mexican Pizza

- 2 pkgs. (10 oz. each) refrigerated pizza crust dough, divided
- 1 - lb. well-trimmed beef top sirloin steak, 1 inch thick, cut into 1½ × ¼-inch-thick strips
- ½ cup chopped onion
- ¾ cup shredded reduced-fat Cheddar cheese (5 g. fat per oz.)
- ½ cup taco sauce
- 1 can (4 oz.) diced green chilies

4 servings

Serving suggestion: Top evenly with 2 cups shredded lettuce, ¾ cup seeded chopped tomato, ¼ cup shredded Cheddar cheese and 3 tablespoons sliced ripe olives.

Per Serving: Calories: 603 • Protein: 43 g. • Carbohydrate: 71 g. • Fat: 13 g. • Cholesterol: 84 mg. • Sodium: 1289 mg. Exchanges: 4½ starch, 3¾ lean meat, ½ vegetable, ½ fat

How to Make Stuffed Mexican Pizza

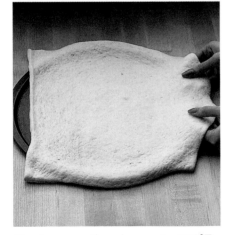

Heat conventional oven to 400°F. Spray 12-inch round pizza pan with nonstick vegetable cooking spray. Place rectangular piece of pizza dough across prepared pan. Stretch dough, leaving 1 inch extending beyond edge of pan. Set aside.

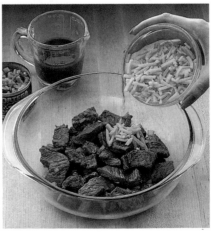

Combine beef strips and onion in 2-quart casserole. Microwave at High for 5 to 7 minutes, or just until meat is only slightly pink, stirring twice. Drain. Add cheese, taco sauce and chilies. Mix well. Spoon meat mixture evenly over crust.

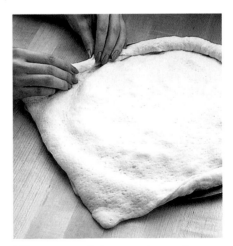

Place remaining rectangular piece of dough over filling, stretching to same size as bottom crust. Roll in edges. Pinch to seal. Bake conventionally for 14 to 17 minutes, or until golden brown.

Stuffed Italian Pizza

2 pkgs. (10 oz. each)
   refrigerated pizza crust
   dough, divided
1-lb. well-trimmed beef
   top sirloin steak, 1 inch
   thick, cut into 1½ × ¼-inch-
   thick strips
½ cup chopped green pepper
½ cup chopped onion
1 can (8 oz.) pizza sauce
1 cup shredded hard farmer
   cheese

4 servings

Heat conventional oven to 400°F.
Spray 12-inch round pizza pan
with nonstick vegetable cooking
spray. Place rectangular piece
of pizza dough across prepared
pan. Stretch dough, leaving 1
inch extending beyond edge of
pan. Set aside.

In 2-quart casserole, combine
beef strips, green pepper and
onion. Microwave at High for 6
to 9 minutes, or just until meat is
only slightly pink, stirring twice.
Drain. Add pizza sauce and
cheese. Mix well.

Spoon meat mixture evenly over
crust. Place remaining rectangular piece of dough over filling,
stretching to same size as bottom crust (opposite). Roll in
edges. Pinch to seal. Bake conventionally for 14 to 17 minutes,
or until golden brown.

Serving suggestion: Top evenly
with ½ cup seeded chopped tomato, ¼ cup snipped fresh basil
leaves and ¼ cup shredded
fresh Parmesan cheese.

Per Serving: Calories: 609 • Protein: 43 g.
• Carbohydrate: 71 g. • Fat: 15 g.
• Cholesterol: 86 mg. • Sodium: 1063 mg.
Exchanges: 4¼ starch, 4 lean meat,
1 vegetable, ½ fat

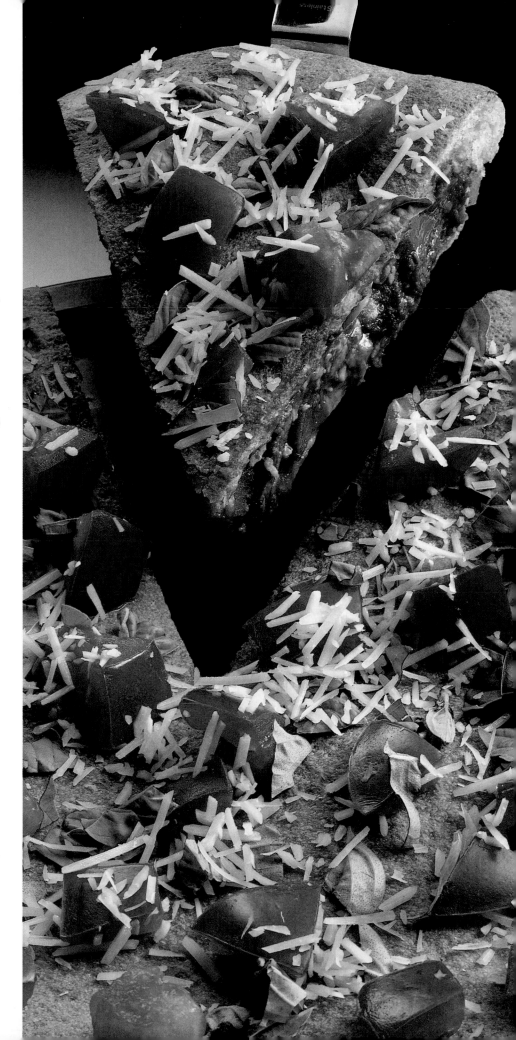

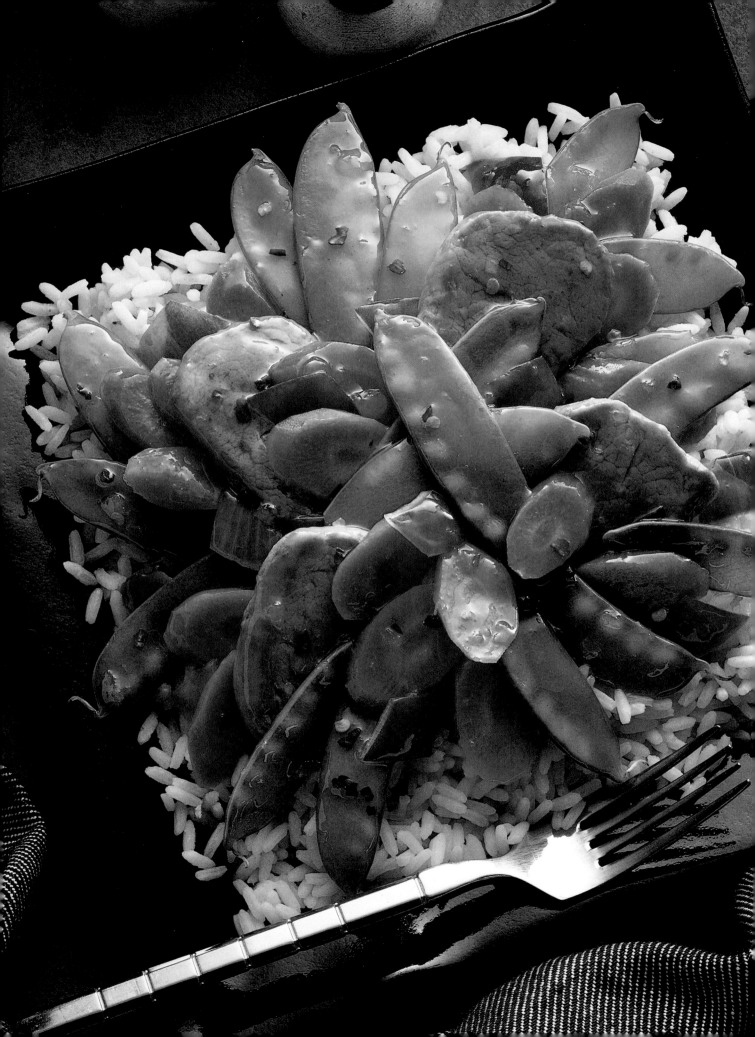

Pork

◀ Spicy Sweet & Sour Pork

1 well-trimmed pork tenderloin (approx. 1 lb.), cut crosswise into 16 pieces
⅛ teaspoon pepper
1 cup sliced carrots
½ cup chopped red onion
6 oz. fresh snow pea pods (2 cups)
¼ cup sweet and sour sauce
¼ teaspoon crushed red pepper flakes

4 servings

Pound pork pieces lightly to ½-inch thickness. Sprinkle evenly with pepper. Spray 12-inch nonstick skillet with nonstick vegetable cooking spray. Heat skillet conventionally over medium-high heat. Add half of pork. Cook for 4 to 6 minutes, or just until meat is no longer pink, turning over once. Remove pork from skillet. Cover to keep warm. Set aside. Repeat with remaining pork.

Place carrots and onion in 3-quart casserole. Cover. Microwave at High for 2 to 4 minutes, or until tender-crisp, stirring once. Stir in pea pods. Re-cover. Microwave at High for 2 to 3 minutes, or until pea pods are tender-crisp, stirring once. Stir in sweet and sour sauce, red pepper flakes and pork. Microwave at High, uncovered, for 1 to 2 minutes, or until hot.

Serving suggestion: Serve with hot cooked rice.

Per Serving: Calories: 193 • Protein: 30 g. • Carbohydrate: 12 g. • Fat: 4 g.
• Cholesterol: 74 mg. • Sodium: 117 mg.
Exchanges: 3 lean meat, 1½ vegetable, ¼ fruit

Broiled Pork & Vegetables

2 cups fresh whole baby carrots (about 12 oz.)
¼ cup water
2 cups halved fresh Brussels sprouts
1 medium zucchini squash, cut lengthwise into quarters, then crosswise into 1½-inch lengths
1 medium yellow summer squash, cut lengthwise into quarters, then crosswise into 1½-inch lengths
2 tablespoons olive oil
2 teaspoons salt-free spicy pepper seasoning, divided
4 well-trimmed boneless pork top loin chops (4 oz. each), 1 inch thick

4 servings

In 2-quart casserole, combine carrots and water. Cover. Microwave at High for 5 minutes. Add Brussels sprouts. Re-cover. Microwave at High for 5 to 8 minutes, or until vegetables are tender-crisp, stirring once. Drain. Add squashes, oil and 1 teaspoon seasoning. Toss to coat. Set aside.

Sprinkle both sides of each chop evenly with remaining 1 teaspoon seasoning. Arrange chops on rack in broiler pan. Arrange vegetables evenly around chops. Place under conventional broiler, with surface of meat 3 to 4 inches from heat. Broil for 10 to 15 minutes, or just until meat is no longer pink, turning chops over and rearranging vegetables once.

Serving suggestion: Serve with steamed new potatoes.

Per Serving: Calories: 300 • Protein: 28 g. • Carbohydrate: 17 g. • Fat: 16 g.
• Cholesterol: 67 mg. • Sodium: 118 mg.
Exchanges: 3 lean meat, 3½ vegetable, 1½ fat

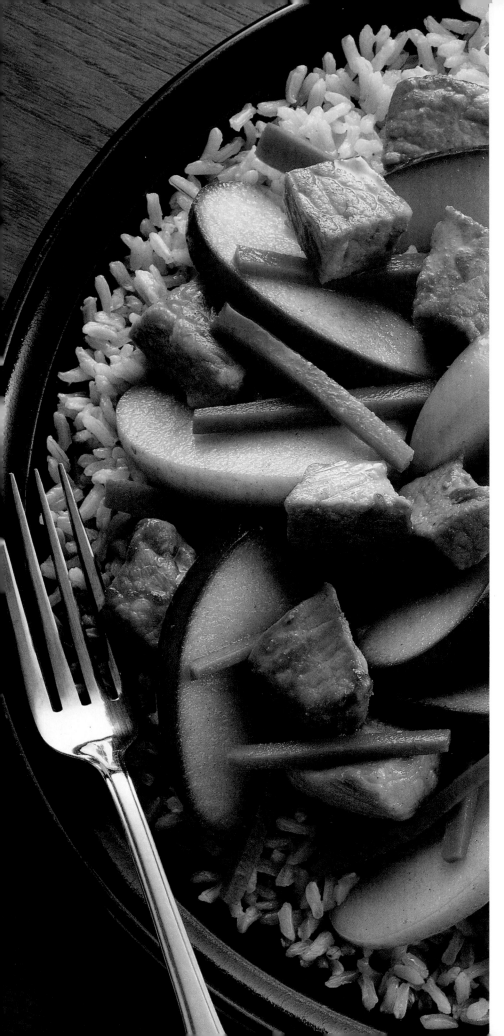

Harvest Spiced Pork & Apples

1- lb. well-trimmed boneless
    pork top loin roast, cut into
    ¾-inch pieces
1 medium Granny Smith
    apple, cored and thinly
    sliced
1 medium Rome apple,
    cored and thinly sliced
1 cup carrot strips
    (2 × ⅛-inch strips)
⅓ cup packed brown sugar
1 tablespoon plus 1
    teaspoon cornstarch
¼ teaspoon ground cinnamon
3 tablespoons cider vinegar

4 servings

Spray 10-inch nonstick skillet with nonstick vegetable cooking spray. Heat skillet conventionally over medium-high heat. Add pork pieces. Cook and stir for 4 to 5 minutes, or just until meat is no longer pink. Remove from heat. Set aside.

In 2-quart casserole, combine apples and carrots. Set aside. In small mixing bowl, combine sugar, cornstarch and cinnamon. Blend in vinegar. Pour over apple mixture. Stir to coat. Microwave at High, uncovered, for 8 to 10 minutes, or until apples and carrots are tender and sauce is thickened and translucent, stirring 2 or 3 times. Add pork. Mix well. Cover. Microwave at High for 1 to 2 minutes, or until hot.

Serving suggestion: Serve with hot cooked rice.

Per Serving: Calories: 325 • Protein: 25 g.
• Carbohydrate: 40 g. • Fat: 9 g.
• Cholesterol: 69 mg. • Sodium: 65 mg.
Exchanges: 3 lean meat, ½ vegetable, 2½ fruit

Chinese Pork ▶ & Pea Pods

8 oz. uncooked vermicelli
4 oz. fresh snow pea pods
    (1½ cups)
1 cup thinly sliced carrots
1-lb. well-trimmed boneless
    pork top loin roast, cut into
    2 × ¼-inch-thick strips
2 tablespoons hoisin sauce
2 tablespoons packed brown
    sugar
1 tablespoon white wine
    vinegar
1 tablespoon reduced-sodium
    soy sauce

4 servings

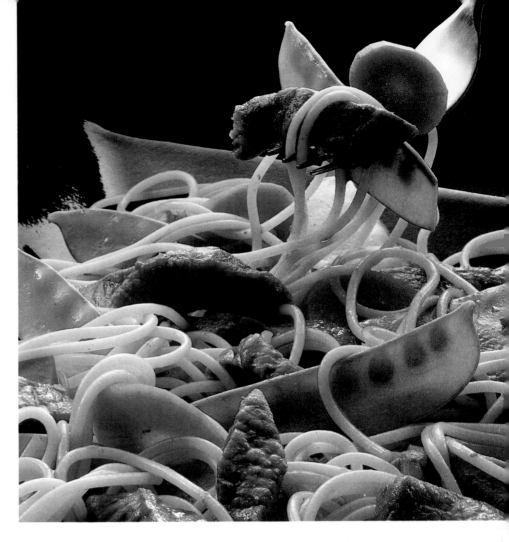

Prepare vermicelli as directed on package. Rinse and drain. Place in large mixing bowl. Set aside. In 2-quart casserole, combine pea pods and carrots. Cover. Microwave at High for 3 to 4 minutes, or until vegetables are tender-crisp. Rinse with cold water. Drain. Add to vermicelli. Set aside.

In same 2-quart casserole, combine pork strips and hoisin sauce. Microwave at High for 5 to 7 minutes, or just until meat is no longer pink, stirring twice. Add to vermicelli mixture. Set aside. In small bowl, combine sugar, vinegar and soy sauce. Microwave at High for 1 to 1½ minutes, or until sugar is dissolved. Add to vermicelli mixture. Toss to coat.

Serving suggestion: Serve with pineapple sorbet.

Per Serving: Calories: 441 • Protein: 33 g.
• Carbohydrate: 57 g. • Fat: 9 g.
• Cholesterol: 69 mg. • Sodium: 471 mg.
Exchanges: 2½ starch, 3 lean meat,
2 vegetable, ½ fruit

Apple-glazed Pork & Sweet Potatoes

2 sweet potatoes (8 oz. each),
    peeled and thinly sliced
¼ cup water
¼ cup apple jelly
2 tablespoons lemon juice
½ teaspoon pumpkin pie
    spice

4 well-trimmed bone-in pork
    center loin or rib chops
    (8 oz. each), 1 inch thick
1 small Rome apple, cored
    and thinly sliced
1 small Granny Smith apple,
    cored and thinly sliced

4 servings

In 2-quart casserole, place sweet potatoes and water. Cover. Microwave at High for 5 to 8 minutes, or until potatoes are tender-crisp, stirring once. Drain. Set aside. In 2-cup measure, combine jelly, juice and pumpkin pie spice. Microwave at High for 2 to 3 minutes, or until jelly is melted, stirring once.

Arrange chops on rack in broiler pan. Arrange sweet potatoes and apples evenly around chops. Brush evenly with half of jelly mixture. Place under conventional broiler, with surface of meat 3 to 4 inches from heat. Broil for 10 to 15 minutes, or just until meat is no longer pink, turning chops over, rearranging vegetables and basting with remaining sauce mixture once.

Serving suggestion: Serve with mixed green salad.

Per Serving: Calories: 357 • Protein: 27 g. • Carbohydrate: 46 g. • Fat: 7 g.
• Cholesterol: 70 mg. • Sodium: 67 mg.
Exchanges: 1½ starch, 3 lean meat, 1½ fruit

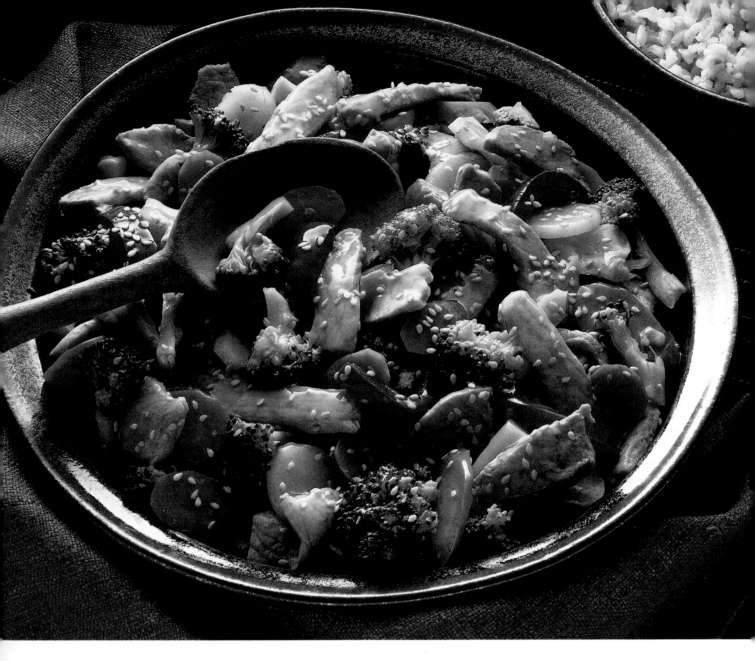

Sesame Pork*

1- lb. well-trimmed boneless
   pork top loin roast, cut into
   2 x ¼-inch-thick strips
1 clove garlic, minced
1 can (14½ oz.) ready-to-serve
   chicken broth
2 tablespoons cornstarch
1 tablespoon reduced-sodium
   soy sauce
1 teaspoon packed brown
   sugar
1 pkg. (16 oz.) frozen broccoli,
   carrots, water chestnuts and
   red pepper
1 tablespoon toasted sesame
   seed

4 servings

Spray 10-inch nonstick skillet with nonstick vegetable cooking spray.
Heat skillet conventionally over medium-high heat. Add pork strips
and garlic. Cook for 5 to 6 minutes, or just until meat is no longer pink.
Set aside. In 2-quart casserole, combine broth, cornstarch, soy sauce
and sugar. Microwave at High for 7 to 9 minutes, or until sauce is
thickened and translucent, stirring twice. Add vegetables and pork.
Mix well. Cover. Microwave at High for 6 to 10 minutes, or until hot,
stirring once. Before serving, sprinkle with sesame seed.

Serving suggestion: Serve with hot cooked rice.

Per Serving: Calories: 261 • Protein: 29 g. • Carbohydrate: 15 g. • Fat: 10 g.
• Cholesterol: 69 mg. • Sodium: 677 mg.
Exchanges: ¼ starch, 3 lean meat, 2½ vegetable

*Recipe not recommended for ovens with less than 600 cooking
watts.

Parmesan Pork & Rice

1- lb. well-trimmed
    boneless pork top loin
    roast, cut into ½-inch
    pieces
1½ cups thinly sliced yellow
    summer squash
1 cup ready-to-serve
    chicken broth
¼ cup dry white wine
½ teaspoon dried basil leaves
1¼ cups uncooked instant rice
½ cup sliced green onions
3 to 4 tablespoons shredded
    fresh Parmesan cheese

4 servings

In 3-quart casserole, microwave
pork pieces at High for 5 to 7
minutes, or just until meat is no
longer pink, stirring twice. Drain.
Add squash, broth, wine and
basil to meat in casserole. Cover.
Microwave at High for 6 to 10 minutes, or until liquid is boiling, stirring once. Stir in rice and onions.
Re-cover. Let stand for 5 minutes.
Sprinkle with Parmesan cheese.

Serving suggestion: Serve with
steamed fresh broccoli spears.

Per Serving: Calories: 325 • Protein: 30 g.
• Carbohydrate: 28 g. • Fat: 10 g.
• Cholesterol: 73 mg. • Sodium: 399 mg.
Exchanges: 1½ starch, 3 lean meat,
1 vegetable

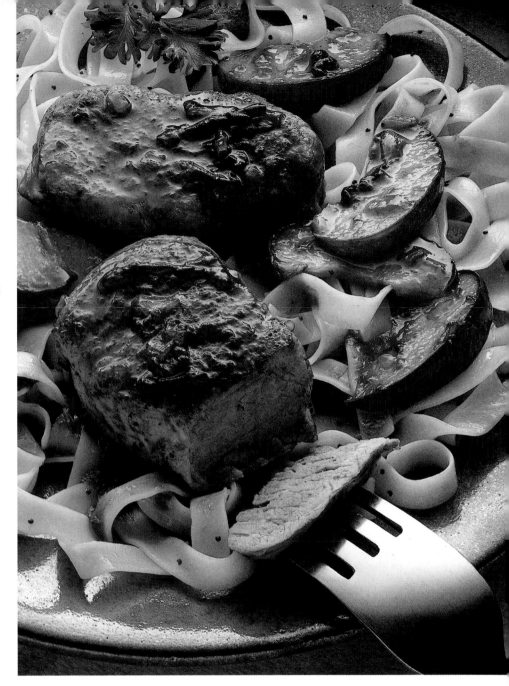

Plum-sauced Pork Medallions ▲

¼ cup chopped onion
½ cup red plum jam
1 tablespoon red wine
    vinegar
1 teaspoon reduced-sodium
    soy sauce
¼ teaspoon ground ginger
2 small plums, each cut into
    8 wedges
1 well-trimmed pork tenderloin
    (approx. 1 lb.), cut crosswise
    into 8 pieces
    Cayenne

4 servings

Place onion in 2-cup measure. Cover with plastic wrap. Microwave
at High for 2 to 3 minutes, or until tender, stirring once. Add jam, vinegar,
soy sauce and ginger. Mix well. Microwave at High, uncovered, for
1½ to 2 minutes, or until jam is melted, stirring once. Add plum wedges.
Set aside. Pound pork pieces lightly to 1-inch thickness. Sprinkle both
sides of each piece lightly with cayenne. Spray 10-inch nonstick skillet
with nonstick vegetable cooking spray. Heat skillet conventionally
over medium-high heat. Add pork. Cook for 6 to 8 minutes, or just
until meat is no longer pink, turning over once. Serve topped with
plum sauce.

Serving suggestion: Serve with hot cooked wide egg noodles
tossed with poppy seed.

Per Serving: Calories: 277 • Protein: 27 g. • Carbohydrate: 32 g. • Fat: 6 g.
• Cholesterol: 80 mg. • Sodium: 110 mg.
Exchanges: 3 lean meat, 1 vegetable, 1¾ fruit

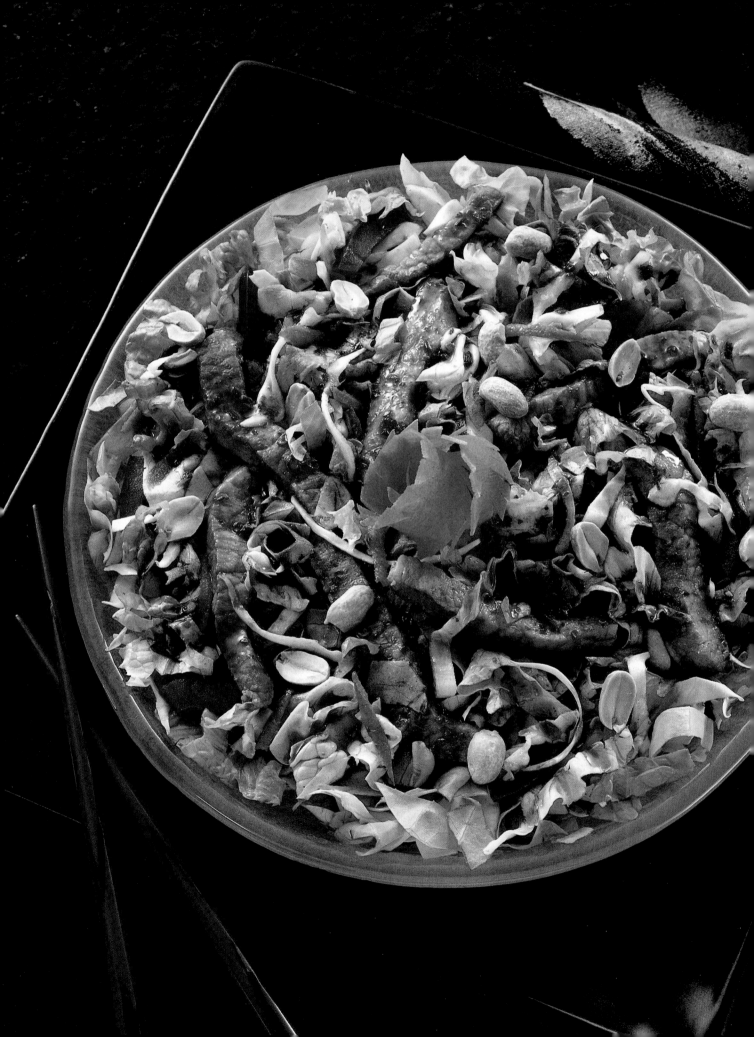

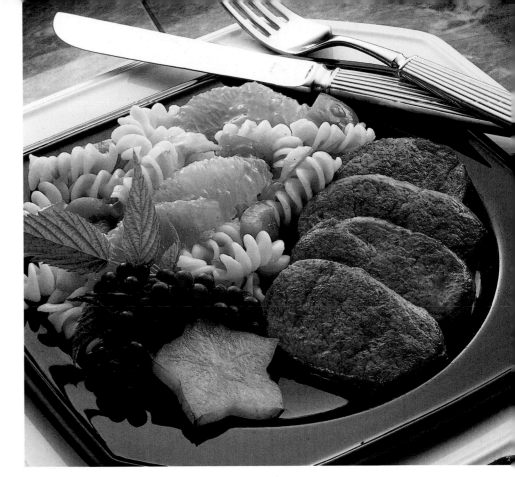

◄ Hot & Spicy Pork Salad

2 tablespoons reduced-sodium soy sauce
1 tablespoon Chinese hot chili sauce with garlic
1 tablespoon vegetable oil
3 cups shredded leaf and Bibb lettuce
1 cup shredded green cabbage
½ cup shredded carrot
½ cup thinly sliced red pepper
1- lb. well-trimmed boneless pork top loin roast, cut into 2 × ¼-inch-thick strips

4 servings

In 1-cup measure, combine soy sauce, chili sauce and oil. Set aside. In medium mixing bowl or salad bowl, combine lettuce, cabbage, carrot and red pepper. Toss to combine. Set aside.

In 2-quart casserole, combine pork strips and 1 tablespoon soy mixture. Microwave at High for 6 to 8 minutes, or just until meat is no longer pink, stirring twice. Drain.

Add meat and remaining soy mixture to lettuce mixture. Toss to coat. Sprinkle with chopped unsalted peanuts, if desired.

Serving suggestion: Serve with fortune cookies.

Per Serving: Calories: 223 • Protein: 26 g.
• Carbohydrate: 5 g. • Fat: 12 g.
• Cholesterol: 69 mg. • Sodium: 385 mg.
Exchanges: 3 lean meat, 1 vegetable, ½ fat

California Pork & Pasta Salad ▲

8 oz. uncooked rotini
1 well-trimmed pork tenderloin (approx. 1 lb.), cut crosswise into 16 pieces
½ teaspoon paprika
1 cup green pepper chunks (1-inch chunks)
⅓ cup white wine vinegar
¼ cup orange marmalade
1 jar (26 oz.) grapefruit and orange sections, drained

4 servings

Prepare rotini as directed on package. Rinse and drain. Set aside. Pound pork pieces lightly to ½-inch thickness. Sprinkle evenly with paprika. Spray 12-inch nonstick skillet with nonstick vegetable cooking spray. Heat skillet conventionally over medium-high heat. Add pork. Cook for 4 to 6 minutes, or just until meat is no longer pink, turning over once. Cover to keep warm. Set aside.

In 1-quart casserole, microwave green pepper at High for 2 to 3 minutes, or until tender-crisp, stirring once. Stir in vinegar and marmalade. Microwave at High for 1 to 2 minutes, or until marmalade is melted; stirring once.

In large mixing bowl or salad bowl, combine rotini and grapefruit and orange sections. Add marmalade mixture. Toss to coat. Serve with pork, or slice pork pieces into ¼-inch strips and toss with rotini mixture.

Serving suggestion: Serve with soft bread sticks.

Per Serving: Calories: 511 • Protein: 33 g. • Carbohydrate: 84 g. • Fat: 5 g.
• Cholesterol: 74 mg. • Sodium: 67 mg.
Exchanges: 2½ starch, 3 lean meat, 3 fruit

Pork Picadillo

1- lb. well-trimmed boneless
    pork top loin roast, cut into
    2 × ⅛-inch-thick strips
1 can (14½ oz.) whole
    tomatoes, undrained and
    cut up
½ cup sliced green onions
½ cup raisins
2 tablespoons tomato paste
2 tablespoons molasses
¼ teaspoon ground ginger
¼ teaspoon salt

4 servings

Place pork strips in 3-quart casserole. Cover. Microwave at High for 4 to 6 minutes, or just until meat is no longer pink, stirring once or twice. Drain. Add remaining ingredients to meat in casserole. Re-cover. Microwave at High for 5 to 7 minutes, or until onions are tender-crisp, stirring once or twice.

Serving suggestion: Serve over hot cooked couscous or rice.

Per Serving: Calories: 279 • Protein: 26 g. • Carbohydrate: 28 g. • Fat: 9 g.
• Cholesterol: 69 mg. • Sodium: 421 mg.
Exchanges: 3 lean meat, 1 vegetable, 1½ fruit

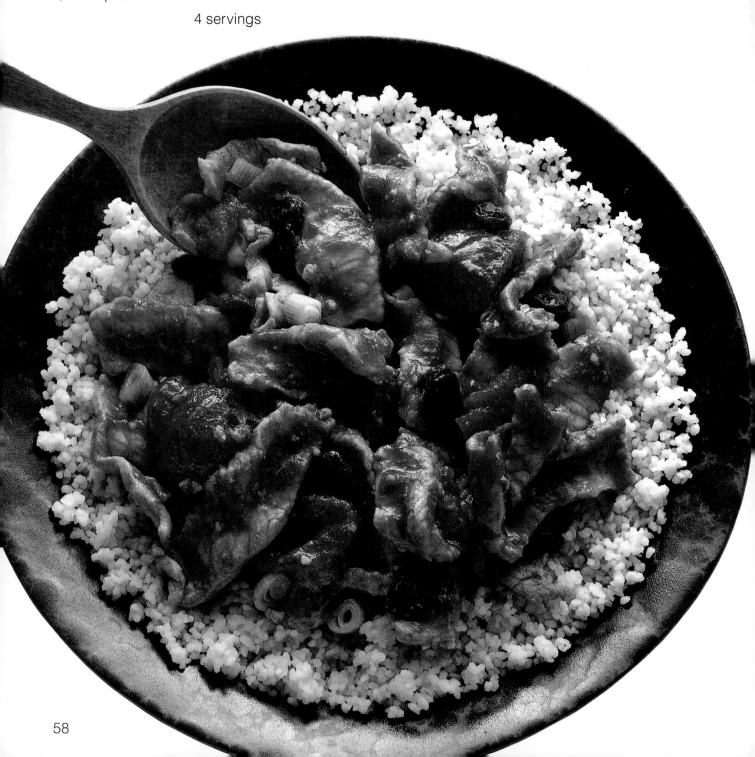

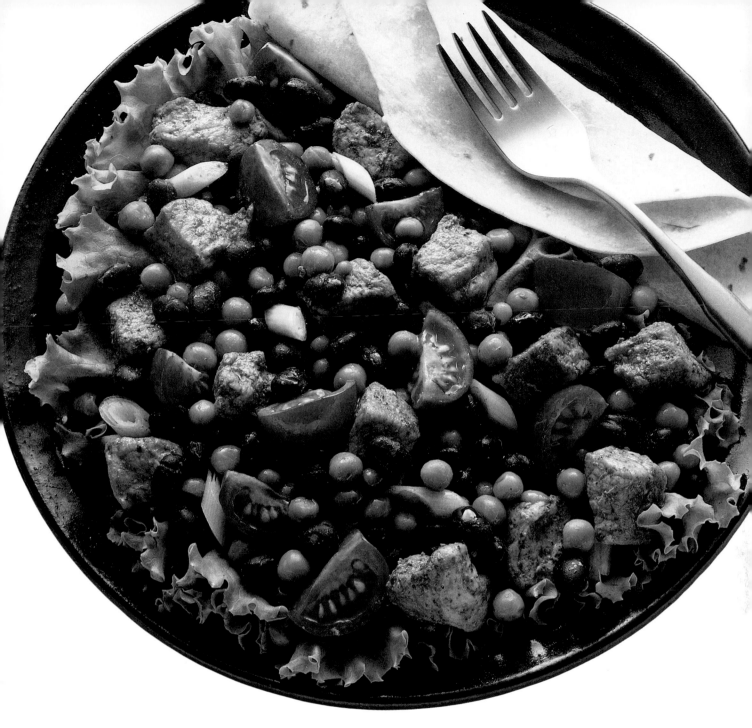

Southwest Pork & Black Bean Salad

1- lb. well-trimmed boneless
   pork top loin roast, cut into
   ¾-inch pieces
1 teaspoon chili powder
½ teaspoon ground cumin
1 can (15 oz.) black beans,
   rinsed and drained
1 cup frozen peas, defrosted
1 cup quartered cherry
   tomatoes
½ cup sliced green onions
1 tablespoon vegetable oil

4 servings

Place pork pieces in 2-quart casserole. Add chili powder and cumin. Stir to coat. Microwave at High for 5 to 6 minutes, or just until meat is no longer pink, stirring once or twice. Drain. Add remaining ingredients to meat in casserole. Mix well. Serve warm.

Serving suggestion: Serve on lettuce-lined plates with warm rolled-up flour tortillas.

Per Serving: Calories: 311 • Protein: 32 g. • Carbohydrate: 19 g. • Fat: 13 g.
• Cholesterol: 69 mg. • Sodium: 231 mg.
Exchanges: 1 starch, 3 lean meat, 1 vegetable, 1 fat

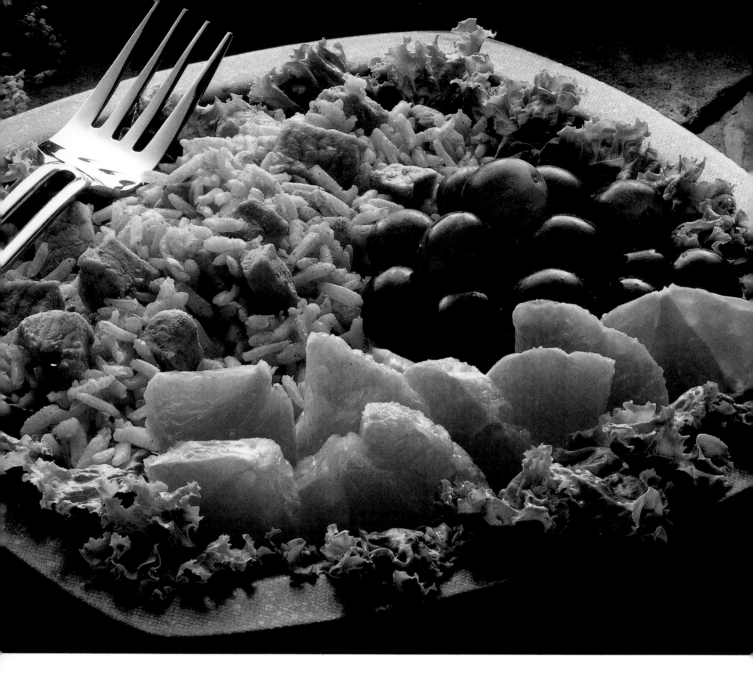

Curried Pork & Brown Rice Salad

1- lb. well-trimmed
    boneless pork top loin
    roast, cut into ½-inch
    pieces
  3 teaspoons curry powder,
    divided
1½ cups uncooked instant
    brown rice
1¼ cups water
  ¼ teaspoon salt
  ¼ cup orange juice
  2 cups seedless red grapes
  2 medium seedless oranges,
    peeled, sliced and cut
    into quarters

4 servings

Place pork pieces in medium mixing bowl. Sprinkle with 1 teaspoon curry powder. Stir to coat. Cover with plastic wrap. Microwave at High for 5 to 7 minutes, or just until meat is no longer pink, stirring twice. Drain. Set aside.

In 2-quart casserole, combine rice, water, salt and remaining 2 teaspoons curry powder. Cover. Microwave at High for 6 to 9 minutes, or until mixture begins to boil. Stir. Let stand, covered, for 5 minutes. Add pork and juice to rice. Mix well. Arrange pork mixture, grapes and oranges evenly on individual serving plates. Serve warm or cold.

Serving suggestion: Serve salad on plates lined with leaf lettuce.

Per Serving: Calories: 365 • Protein: 28 g. • Carbohydrate: 47 g. • Fat: 10 g.
• Cholesterol: 69 mg. • Sodium: 201 mg.
Exchanges: 1½ starch, 3 lean meat, 1⅔ fruit

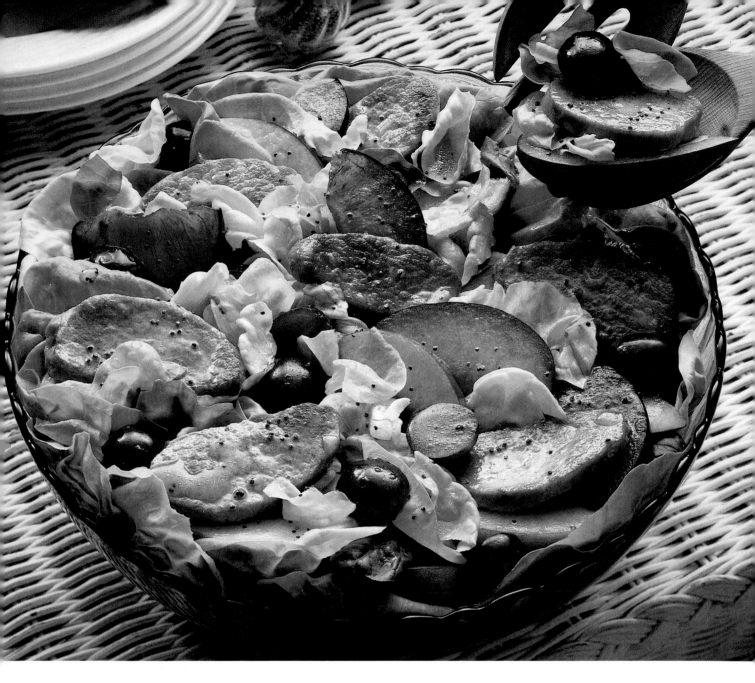

Fruited Pork Salad

4 cups torn fresh greens
(spinach or Bibb lettuce)
2 cups sliced fresh fruit
(nectarines, plums and
grapes)
1 well-trimmed pork tenderloin
(approx. 1 lb.), cut crosswise
into 20 pieces
3 tablespoons orange juice
2 tablespoons red wine
vinegar
2 tablespoons vegetable oil
1 tablespoon honey
1 teaspoon poppy seed

4 servings

In large mixing bowl or salad bowl, combine greens and fruit. Set aside. Spray 12-inch nonstick skillet with nonstick vegetable cooking spray. Heat skillet conventionally over medium-high heat. Add half of the pork pieces. Cook for 3 to 4 minutes, or just until meat is no longer pink, turning over once. Remove pork from skillet. Set aside. Repeat with remaining pork. Add pork to greens. In 2-cup measure, combine remaining ingredients. Microwave at High for 2 to 3 minutes, or until hot, stirring once. Add dressing to greens. Toss to coat.

Serving suggestion: Serve with warm crescent rolls.

Per Serving: Calories: 291 • Protein: 28 g. • Carbohydrate: 18 g. • Fat: 13 g.
• Cholesterol: 80 mg. • Sodium: 80 mg.
Exchanges: 3 lean meat, ½ vegetable, 1 fruit, 1 fat

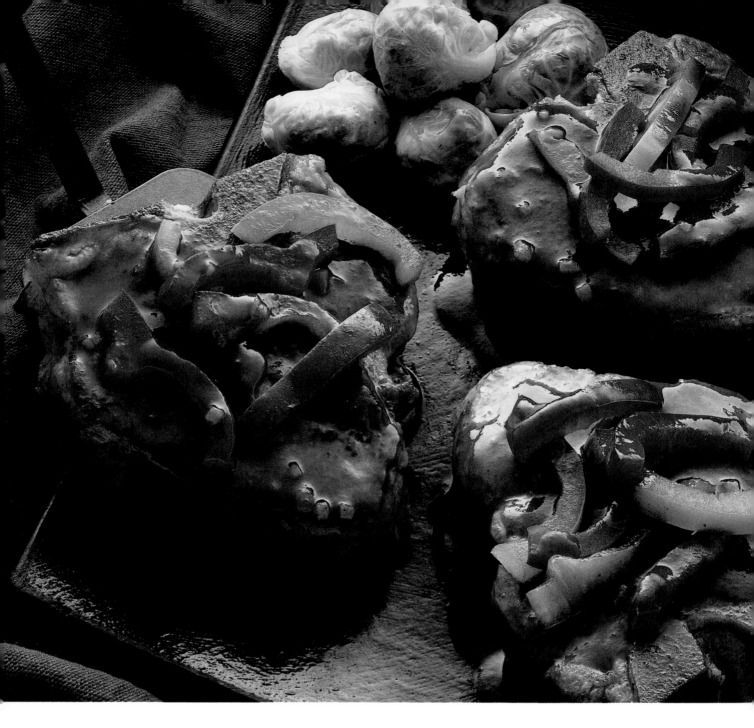

Spicy Gingered Pork Chops

½ cup barbecue sauce
¼ cup honey
2 tablespoons reduced-sodium
   soy sauce
1 tablespoon lemon juice
1 teaspoon ground ginger
1 clove garlic, minced
4 well-trimmed bone-in pork
   center loin or rib chops
   (8 oz. each), 1 inch thick
1 cup green and red pepper
   strips (2 × ¼-inch strips)

4 servings

In 2-cup measure, combine barbecue sauce, honey, soy sauce, juice, ginger and garlic. Set aside. Spray 10-inch nonstick skillet with nonstick vegetable cooking spray. Heat skillet conventionally over medium-high heat. Add pork chops. Cook for 5 to 6 minutes, or just until browned on both sides. Arrange chops in 10-inch square casserole. Pour sauce mixture over chops. Sprinkle with pepper strips. Cover. Microwave at 70% (Medium High) for 10 to 12 minutes, or just until meat is no longer pink, turning chops over and rearranging once.

Serving suggestion: Serve with lightly buttered Brussels sprouts.

Per Serving: Calories: 285 • Protein: 29 g. • Carbohydrate: 24 g. • Fat: 10 g.
• Cholesterol: 78 mg. • Sodium: 631 mg.
Exchanges: 3 lean meat, ¼ vegetable, 1½ fruit

62

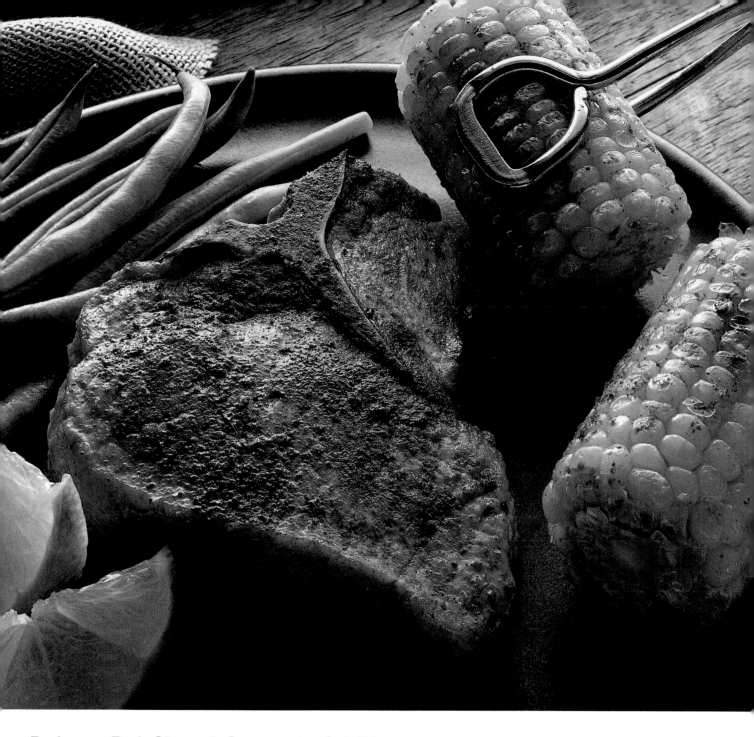

Barbecue Pork Chops & Corn on the Cob Dinner

6 miniature (2½ to 3-inch)
    ears frozen corn on the cob
¼ cup water
4 well-trimmed bone-in pork
    center loin or rib chops
    (8 oz. each), 1 inch thick
1 tablespoon barbecue
    seasoning
1 lime, cut into 8 wedges

4 servings

Place corn and water in 8-inch square baking dish. Cover with plastic wrap. Microwave at High for 8½ to 14 minutes, or until hot, rearranging twice. Sprinkle both sides of pork chops and corn lightly with barbecue seasoning. Set corn aside. Arrange chops on rack in broiler pan. Place under conventional broiler, with surface of meat 3 to 4 inches from heat. Broil for 10 minutes. Turn chops over. Arrange corn around chops. Continue broiling for 3 to 7 minutes, or just until meat is no longer pink and corn is lightly browned. Serve with lime wedges.

Serving suggestion: Serve with steamed green beans.

Per Serving: Calories: 277 • Protein: 30 g. • Carbohydrate: 25 g. • Fat: 7 g.
• Cholesterol: 68 mg. • Sodium: 111 mg.
Exchanges: 1½ starch, 3 lean meat

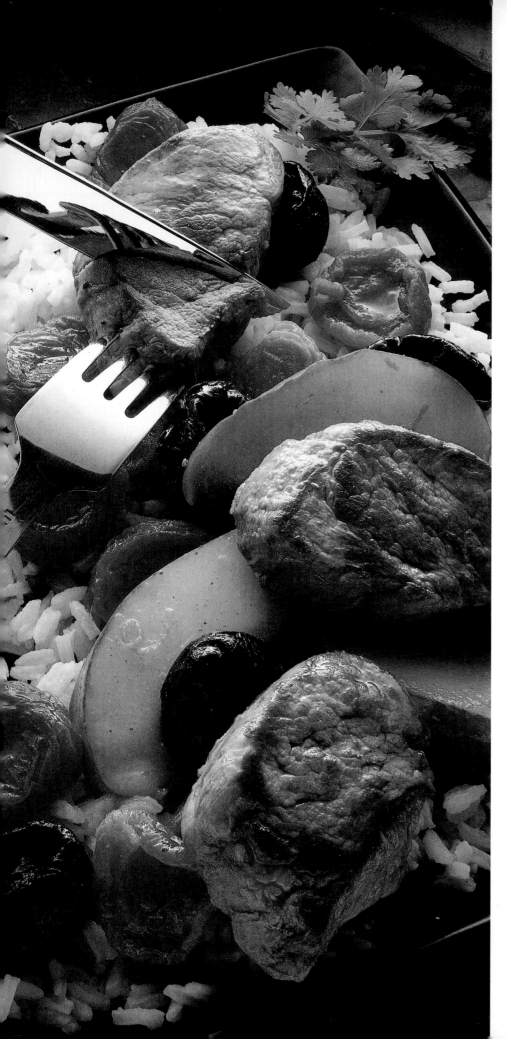

Pork Tenderloin with Curried Mixed Fruits

2 well-trimmed pork tenderloins (approx. ¾ lb. each), each cut crosswise into 9 pieces
1 pkg. (6 oz.) dried apricots
1 cup pitted prunes
1 teaspoon curry powder
1 teaspoon cornstarch
¾ cup orange juice
1 large pear, cored and sliced
½ teaspoon grated orange peel

4 to 6 servings

Pound pork pieces lightly to ¾-inch thickness. Sprinkle evenly with salt and pepper, if desired. Set aside. In 2-quart casserole, combine apricots and prunes. Sprinkle with curry powder and cornstarch. Toss to coat. Blend in juice. Add pear slices and orange peel. Mix well. Cover. Microwave at High for 8 to 10 minutes, or until pear slices are tender and sauce is thickened and translucent, stirring twice. Cover to keep warm. Set aside.

Spray 12-inch nonstick skillet with nonstick vegetable cooking spray. Heat skillet conventionally over medium-high heat. Add half of the pork. Cook for 4 to 6 minutes, or just until meat is no longer pink, turning over once. Remove pork from skillet. Cover to keep warm. Set aside. Repeat with remaining pork. Spoon curried fruit mixture evenly onto individual serving plates. Top evenly with pork.

Serving suggestion: Serve with hot cooked rice.

Per Serving: Calories: 384 • Protein: 34 g. • Carbohydrate: 52 g. • Fat: 7 g. • Cholesterol: 96 mg. • Sodium: 72 mg. Exchanges: 3 lean meat, 3½ fruit

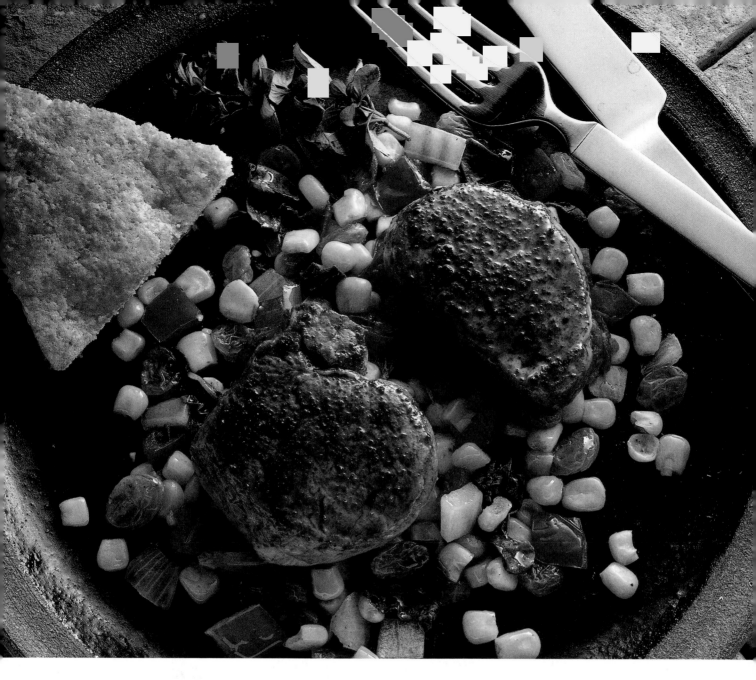

Pork Tenderloin with Sweet Corn Chutney

1 well-trimmed pork tenderloin (approx. 1 lb.), cut crosswise into 12 pieces
½ teaspoon chili powder, divided
1 cup frozen corn
1 cup seeded chopped tomato
½ cup chopped red onion
½ cup golden raisins
½ teaspoon dried oregano leaves
2 cups torn fresh spinach leaves

4 servings

Pound pork pieces lightly to ¾-inch thickness. Sprinkle evenly with ¼ teaspoon chili powder. Spray 12-inch nonstick skillet with nonstick vegetable cooking spray. Heat skillet conventionally over medium-high heat. Add pork. Cook for 4 to 6 minutes, or just until meat is no longer pink, turning over once. Cover to keep warm. Set aside. In 2-quart casserole, combine corn, tomato, onion, raisins, oregano and remaining ¼ teaspoon chili powder. Cover. Microwave at High for 4 to 7 minutes, or until onion is tender and mixture is hot. Stir in spinach. Re-cover. Microwave at High for 1 to 1½ minutes, or until spinach is wilted. Spoon corn chutney evenly onto individual serving plates. Top evenly with pork.

Serving suggestion: Serve with jalapeño corn bread and tossed salad.

Per Serving: Calories: 252 • Protein: 27 g. • Carbohydrate: 28 g. • Fat: 5 g.
• Cholesterol: 74 mg. • Sodium: 89 mg.
Exchanges: ½ starch, 3 lean meat, 1 vegetable, 1 fruit

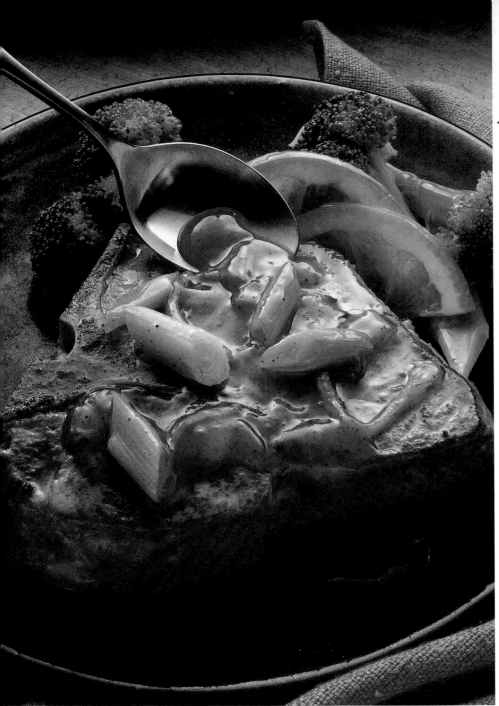

◄ Sweet & Zesty Orange Pork Chops

    4 well-trimmed bone-in pork
        center loin or rib chops
        (8 oz. each), 1 inch thick
    ½ cup sliced green onions
        (½-inch slices)
    ½ cup orange juice
    ¼ cup orange marmalade
    1 tablespoon cornstarch
    ¼ teaspoon salt
    ¼ teaspoon cayenne

4 servings

Spray 12-inch nonstick skillet with nonstick vegetable cooking spray. Heat skillet conventionally over medium-high heat. Add pork chops. Cook for 5 to 6 minutes, or just until browned on both sides. Arrange chops in 10-inch square casserole. Set aside. In 2-cup measure, combine remaining ingredients. Spoon over chops. Cover. Microwave at 70% (Medium High) for 10 to 12 minutes, or just until meat is no longer pink and sauce is thickened, rearranging chops and stirring sauce twice.

Serving suggestion: Serve with steamed fresh broccoli spears.

Per Serving: Calories: 259 • Protein: 28 g.
• Carbohydrate: 20 g. • Fat: 9 g.
• Cholesterol: 78 mg. • Sodium: 212 mg.
Exchanges: 3 lean meat, 1⅓ fruit

Honey & Soy Glazed Pork Chops

    2 tablespoons finely
        chopped onion
    1 clove garlic, minced
    1 teaspoon water
    ¼ cup catsup
    2 tablespoons honey
    1 tablespoon reduced-sodium
        soy sauce
    ½ teaspoon ground ginger
    4 well-trimmed bone-in pork
        center loin or rib chops
        (8 oz. each), 1 inch thick

4 servings

In 4-cup measure, combine onion, garlic and water. Cover with plastic wrap. Microwave at High for 1 to 2 minutes, or until onion is tender, stirring once. Add remaining ingredients, except pork chops. Mix well. Microwave at High, uncovered, for 2 to 3 minutes, or until hot. Arrange chops on rack in broiler pan. Brush with half of honey-soy mixture. Place chops under conventional broiler, with surface of meat 3 to 4 inches from heat. Broil for 10 to 15 minutes, or just until meat is no longer pink, turning chops over and brushing with remaining sauce mixture once.

Serving suggestion: Serve with sweet corn and cucumber salad.

Per Serving: Calories: 228 • Protein: 26 g. • Carbohydrate: 14 g. • Fat: 7 g.
• Cholesterol: 70 mg. • Sodium: 380 mg.
Exchanges: 3 lean meat, 1 fruit

Pork Tenderloin with Garlic Tomato Sauce

¼ cup chopped onion
¾ cup ready-to-serve chicken broth
3 tablespoons garlic-flavored red wine vinegar
2 tablespoons tomato paste
2 teaspoons cornstarch
2 teaspoons sugar
1 well-trimmed pork tenderloin (approx. 1 lb.), cut crosswise into 8 pieces

4 servings

Place onion in 4-cup measure. Cover with plastic wrap. Microwave at High for 2 to 3 minutes, or until tender, stirring once. Add remaining ingredients, except pork pieces. Mix well. Microwave at High, uncovered, for 3 to 4 minutes, or until sauce is thickened and translucent, stirring once. Set aside.

Pound pork pieces lightly to 1-inch thickness. Spray 10-inch nonstick skillet with nonstick vegetable cooking spray. Heat skillet conventionally over medium-high heat. Add pork. Cook for 4 to 6 minutes, or just until meat is no longer pink, turning over once. Spoon sauce evenly over pork.

Serving suggestion: Serve with hot cooked rice and steamed whole green beans.

Per Serving: Calories: 168 • Protein: 25 g.
• Carbohydrate: 6 g. • Fat: 4 g.
• Cholesterol: 74 mg. • Sodium: 307 mg.
Exchanges: 3 lean meat, 1 vegetable

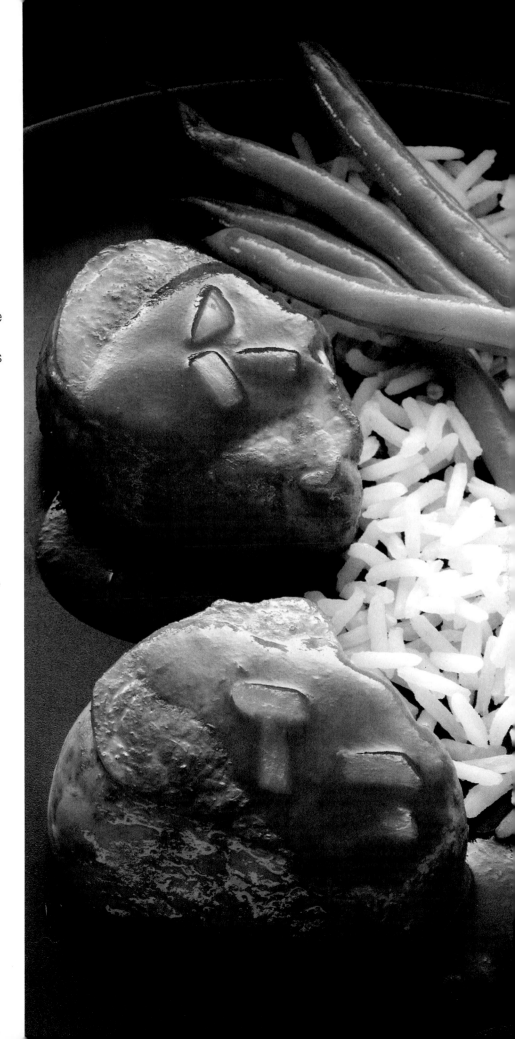

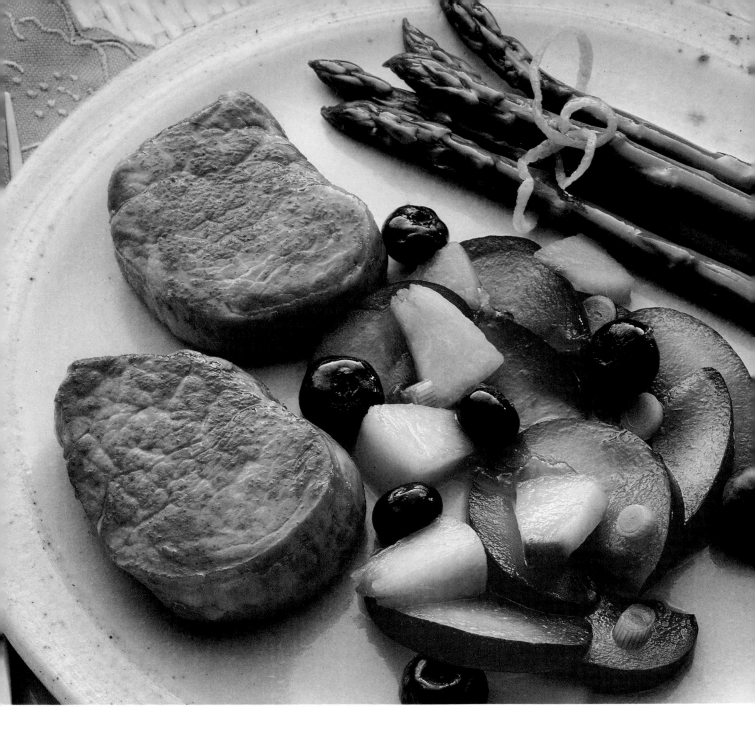

Pork Tenderloin with Summer Fruit Salsa

  1 medium fresh peach, peeled
     and chopped
  2 small fresh plums, thinly sliced
 ½ cup sliced green onions or
     chopped red onion
 ½ cup fresh blueberries
 ¼ cup peach preserves
  1 well-trimmed pork tenderloin
     (approx. 1 lb.), cut
     crosswise into 8 pieces

4 servings

In small mixing bowl, combine peach, plums, onions and blueberries. Set aside. In 1-cup measure, microwave preserves at High for 1½ to 2 minutes, or until melted, stirring once. Pour over fruit mixture. Toss to coat. Set salsa aside. Pound pork pieces lightly to 1-inch thickness. Spray 10-inch nonstick skillet with nonstick vegetable cooking spray. Heat skillet conventionally over medium-high heat. Add pork. Cook for 4 to 6 minutes, or just until meat is no longer pink, turning over once. Serve with salsa.

Serving suggestion: Serve with steamed fresh asparagus spears and crusty French bread.

Per Serving: Calories: 250 • Protein: 25 g. • Carbohydrate: 28 g. • Fat: 5 g.
• Cholesterol: 74 mg. • Sodium: 61 mg.
Exchanges: 3 lean meat, 2 fruit

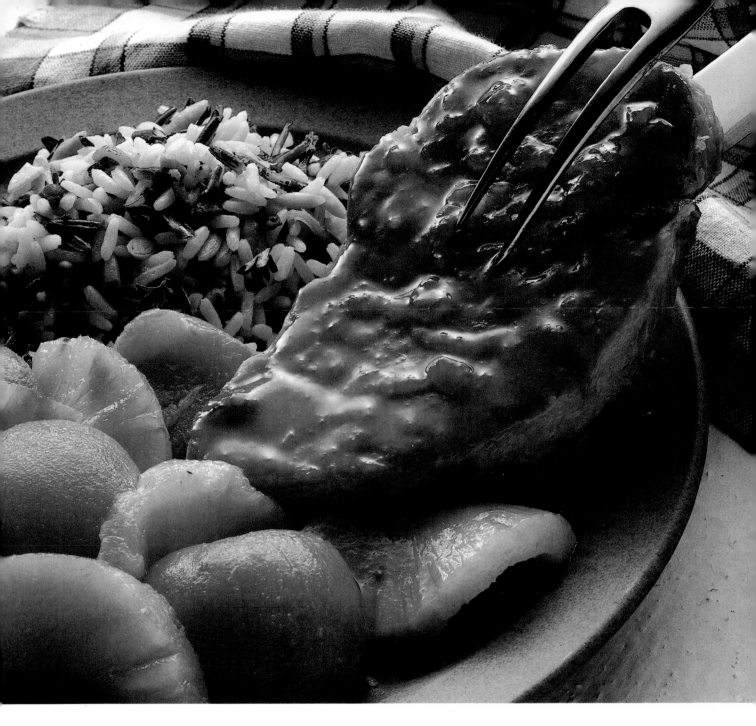

Broiled Fruited Ham Steak

1½-lb. well-trimmed fully
     cooked bone-in ham
     steak, ¾ inch thick
1 can (8¼ oz.) pineapple
     slices in juice, drained
     (reserve ¼ cup juice)
1 can (16 oz.) apricot halves,
     rinsed and drained
¼ cup apricot preserves
2 teaspoons Dijon mustard
2 teaspoons cider vinegar

4 servings

Place ham on rack in broiler pan. Cut pineapple slices in half. Arrange pineapple and apricots evenly around ham steak. In 2-cup measure, combine remaining ingredients, except reserved juice. Microwave at High for 2 to 3 minutes, or until preserves are melted, stirring once. Brush ham steak with half of mixture. Brush pineapple and apricots with half of reserved juice. Place ham steak under conventional broiler with surface of meat 3 to 4 inches from heat. Broil for 10 to 11 minutes, or until hot, turning ham over and basting ham with remaining mixture and fruit with remaining juice once.

Serving suggestion: Serve with wild rice pilaf.

Per Serving: Calories: 242 • Protein: 22 g. • Carbohydrate: 28 g. • Fat: 5 g.
• Cholesterol: 49 mg. • Sodium: 1428 mg.
Exchanges: 3 lean meat, 2 fruit

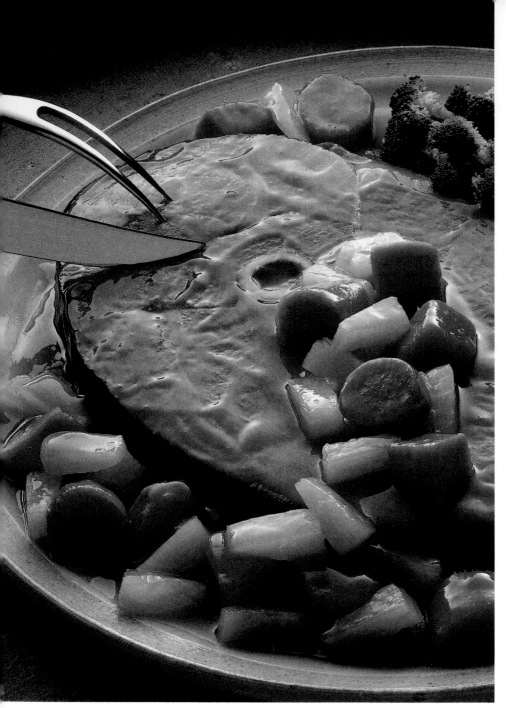

Ham & Tomato Salad Sandwiches

¾ lb. shaved fully cooked
    boneless ham, chopped
1 cup seeded chopped
    tomato
¼ cup sliced green onions
¼ cup reduced-calorie
    mayonnaise
1 tablespoon Dijon mustard
8 slices reduced-calorie
    whole wheat bread, toasted

4 servings

In medium mixing bowl, combine all ingredients, except
toast. Microwave at High for 3
to 4 minutes, or until hot, stirring once. Spoon ham mixture
evenly onto 4 toast slices. Top
with remaining toast slices.

Serving suggestion: Garnish
sandwiches with leaf lettuce or
fresh spinach leaves.

Per Serving: Calories: 291 • Protein: 23 g.
• Carbohydrate: 26 g. • Fat: 11 g.
• Cholesterol: 51 mg. • Sodium: 1513 mg.
Exchanges: 1 starch, 3 lean meat,
2 vegetable, ¼ fat

Pineapple & Rum Sauced Ham Steak* ▲

1½-lb. well-trimmed fully
    cooked bone-in ham
    steak, ¾ inch thick
1 can (18 oz.) sweet
    potatoes, drained and cut
    into 1-inch chunks
1 can (8 oz.) pineapple
    tidbits in juice, undrained
¾ cup packed brown sugar
2 tablespoons dark rum
1 tablespoon cornstarch
1 teaspoon dry mustard

4 servings

Place ham steak in 10-inch square casserole. Set aside. In medium
mixing bowl, combine remaining ingredients. Pour sauce evenly over
ham steak. Cover. Microwave at High for 15 to 17 minutes, or until
sauce is thickened and translucent and ham is hot, stirring sauce
twice and rotating dish once.

Serving suggestion: Serve with steamed broccoli flowerets and
saffron rice.

Per Serving: Calories: 341 • Protein: 23 g. • Carbohydrate: 52 g. • Fat: 5 g.
• Cholesterol: 49 mg. • Sodium: 1427 mg.
Exchanges: 1 starch, 3 lean meat, 2½ fruit

*Recipe not recommended for ovens with less than 600 cooking
watts.

Jazzed Up Ham & Beans ▶

¾ cup chopped onion, divided
¾ cup chopped green pepper,
   divided
1 pkg. (9 oz.) frozen lima beans
¾ lb. fully cooked boneless
   ham, cut into 1½ × ¼-inch-
   thick strips
1 can (16 oz.) baked beans
1 cup seeded chopped
   tomato

4 servings

In 3-quart casserole, combine
½ cup onion, ½ cup green pepper and the lima beans. Cover.
Microwave at High for 4 to 6 minutes, or until vegetables are
tender-crisp, stirring once. Stir
in ham strips and baked beans.
Re-cover. Microwave at High
for 6 to 9 minutes, or until hot,
stirring once. Before serving,
sprinkle with tomato and remaining
¼ cup onion and green pepper.

Serving suggestion: Serve with
warm soft bread sticks.

Per Serving: Calories: 325 • Protein: 29 g.
• Carbohydrate: 41 g. • Fat: 6 g.
• Cholesterol: 53 mg. • Sodium: 1564 mg.
Exchanges: 2½ starch, 3 lean meat,
½ vegetable

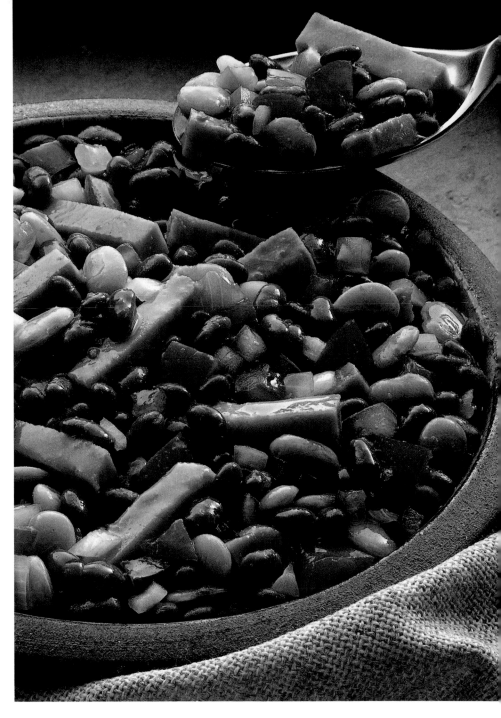

Caraway Ham & Cabbage Stir-fry

4 cups coarsely chopped red
   and green cabbage
1 cup carrot strips (2 ×¼-inch
   strips)
½ cup diagonally sliced green
   onions (½-inch lengths)
¼ cup packed brown sugar
2 tablespoons white vinegar
½ teaspoon caraway seed
¾ lb. fully cooked boneless
   ham, cut into thin strips

4 servings

In 3-quart casserole, combine cabbage, carrots, onions, sugar, vinegar
and caraway seed. Microwave at High, uncovered, for 5 to 8 minutes,
or until vegetables are tender-crisp, stirring twice. Add ham strips.
Microwave at High for 1½ to 3 minutes, or until hot, stirring once.

Serving suggestion: Serve with dark rye or pumpernickel bread.

Per Serving: Calories: 209 • Protein: 19 g. • Carbohydrate: 23 g. • Fat: 5 g.
• Cholesterol: 45 mg. • Sodium: 1049 mg.
Exchanges: 3 lean meat, 1½ vegetable, 1 fruit

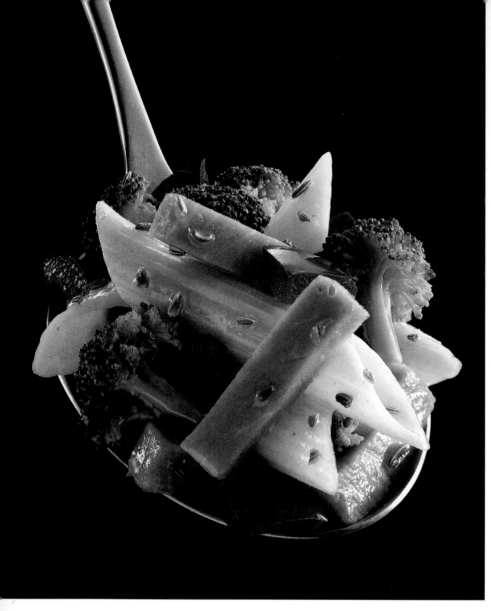

◄ Warm Pasta & Ham Salad

- 8 oz. uncooked mostaccioli
- 2 cups fresh broccoli flowerets
- 1 cup coarsely chopped red pepper
- 2 tablespoons olive oil
- 2 tablespoons cider vinegar
- ½ teaspoon fennel seed, crushed
- ¼ teaspoon salt
- ¾ lb. fully cooked boneless ham, cut into 1 × ¼-inch-thick strips

4 servings

Cook mostaccioli as directed on package. Rinse and drain. Set aside. Place broccoli in 2-quart casserole. Cover. Microwave at High for 3 to 4 minutes, or until tender-crisp, stirring once. Add red pepper. Mix well. Re-cover. Microwave at High for 2 to 3 minutes, or until vegetables are tender, stirring once. Drain. Set aside.

In large mixing bowl or salad bowl, combine oil, vinegar, fennel seed and salt. Add ham strips, mostaccioli and vegetables. Toss to coat. Serve salad warm.

Serving suggestion: Serve with crusty French bread.

Per Serving: Calories: 421 • Protein: 27 g.
• Carbohydrate: 49 g. • Fat: 13 g.
• Cholesterol: 45 mg. • Sodium: 1179 mg.
Exchanges: 2½ starch, 3 lean meat, 1 fat

Black-eyed Peas & Ham Salad

- 2 tablespoons vegetable oil
- 2 tablespoons red wine vinegar
- 2 tablespoons low-calorie mayonnaise or salad dressing
- ¼ teaspoon salt
- ⅛ teaspoon cayenne

- 1 small green pepper, cut into ½-inch chunks
- 1 can (16 oz.) black-eyed peas, rinsed and drained
- ¾ lb. fully cooked boneless ham, cut into 1½ × ½-inch-thick strips

4 servings

In medium mixing bowl, combine oil, vinegar, mayonnaise, salt and cayenne. Set aside. Place green pepper in 1-quart casserole. Cover. Microwave at High for 2 to 3 minutes, or until color brightens and peppers are hot. Rinse with cold water. Drain. Add green pepper, peas and ham strips to dressing mixture. Toss to coat. Serve on bed of lettuce and garnish with tomato wedges, if desired.

Serving suggestion: Serve with warm corn muffins.

Per Serving: Calories: 301 • Protein: 24 g. • Carbohydrate: 19 g. • Fat: 14 g.
• Cholesterol: 48 mg. • Sodium: 1539 mg.
Exchanges: 1¼ starch, 3 lean meat, 1 fat

Light & Easy ▶
Focaccia Pizza*

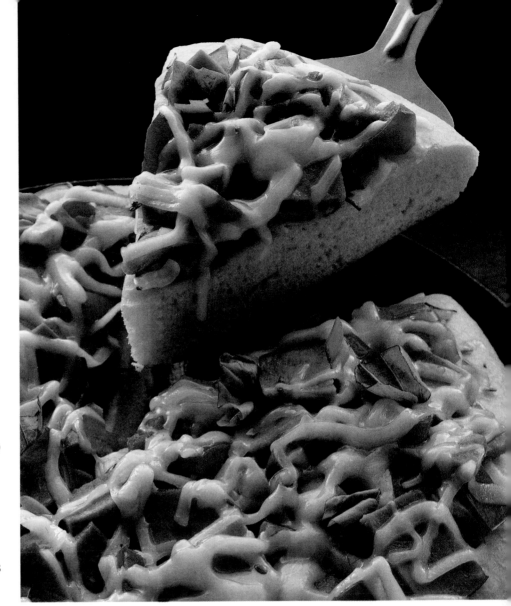

½ lb. Canadian-style bacon
    slices, chopped
1 cup seeded chopped tomato
⅓ cup sliced green onions
2 oz. farmer cheese,
    shredded (½ cup)
6 to 10 fresh basil leaves,
    snipped
1 Focaccia loaf (1 lb.)

4 servings

In small mixing bowl, combine
bacon, tomato, onions, cheese
and basil. Place Focaccia loaf
on 12-inch platter. Top evenly with
bacon mixture.

Microwave at 70% (Medium
High) for 5 to 6 minutes, or just
until cheese begins to melt and
bread is warm, rotating once.

Serving suggestion: Serve with
Bibb lettuce and spinach salad.

Per Serving: Calories: 422 • Protein: 28 g.
• Carbohydrate: 53 g. • Fat: 12 g.
• Cholesterol: 39 mg. • Sodium: 1469 mg.
Exchanges: 3½ starch, 2½ lean meat, 1 fat

*Recipe not recommended for
ovens with less than 600 cooking watts.

Spicy Canadian-style Bacon & Corn Salad

1 pkg. (3 oz.) Ramen soup
    mix (discard seasoning
    packet)
1 pkg. (16 oz.) frozen corn,
    red and green pepper
¾ lb. Canadian-style bacon
    slices, cut into quarters

2 tablespoons canned
    chopped green chilies or
    canned diced jalapeño
    peppers
½ cup fat-free Italian dressing
1 tablespoon sugar
¼ teaspoon celery seed

4 servings

Prepare noodles as directed on package. Rinse and drain. Place
in large mixing bowl or salad bowl. Set aside. Place corn mixture
in 2-quart casserole. Cover. Microwave at High for 7 to 10 minutes,
or until hot, stirring twice. Drain. Add corn, bacon and chilies to
noodles. Mix well. In 1-cup measure, combine remaining ingredients.
Pour over salad mixture. Toss to coat.

Serving suggestion: Serve with herbed bread sticks.

Per Serving: Calories: 346 • Protein: 23 g. • Carbohydrate: 40 g. • Fat: 11 g.
• Cholesterol: 43 mg. • Sodium: 1780 mg.
Exchanges: 2 starch, 3 lean meat, 1 vegetable, ½ fat

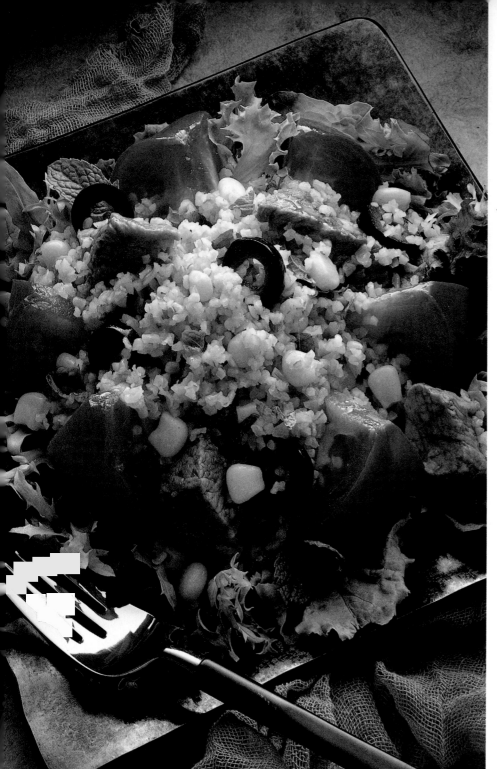

Lamb & Veal

◄ Lebanese Lamb & Bulgur Salad

    1 cup uncooked bulgur
    1- lb. well-trimmed boneless
        lamb leg roast, cut into
        ¾-inch pieces
    1 cup frozen corn
    ⅓ cup fresh mint leaves
    ¼ cup sliced black olives
    3 tablespoons lemon juice
    1 tablespoon vegetable oil
    ½ teaspoon garlic salt

4 servings

Place bulgur in medium mixing bowl. Cover with boiling water. Set aside. In 2-quart casserole, microwave lamb pieces at High, uncovered, for 3 to 7 minutes, or just until meat is only slightly pink, stirring twice. Add corn. Mix well. Microwave at High for 1 to 2 minutes, or until mixture is hot, stirring once. Drain. Set aside. Drain bulgur. Add bulgur and remaining ingredients to meat mixture. Mix well.

Serving suggestion: Serve salad warm in hollowed-out tomato shells.

Per Serving: Calories: 351 • Protein: 29 g. • Carbohydrate: 37 g. • Fat: 11 g. • Cholesterol: 75 mg. • Sodium: 385 mg. Exchanges: 2 starch, 3 lean meat, 1 vegetable, ½ fat

Jalapeño-glazed Lamb Chops

    ½ cup jalapeño jelly
    8 well-trimmed lamb rib or
        loin chops (approx. 6 oz.
        each), 1 inch thick

4 servings

In 2-cup measure, microwave jelly at High for 2 to 3 minutes, or until melted, stirring once. Arrange chops on rack in broiler pan. Brush evenly with half of jelly. Place under conventional broiler, with surface of meat 3 to 4 inches from heat. Broil for 7 to 11 minutes, or until desired doneness, turning chops over and brushing with remaining jelly once.

Serving suggestion: Serve with rice pilaf.

Per Serving: Calories: 316 • Protein: 25 g. • Carbohydrate: 26 g. • Fat: 12 g. • Cholesterol: 83 mg. • Sodium: 83 mg. Exchanges: 3 lean meat, 1¾ fruit, ½ fat

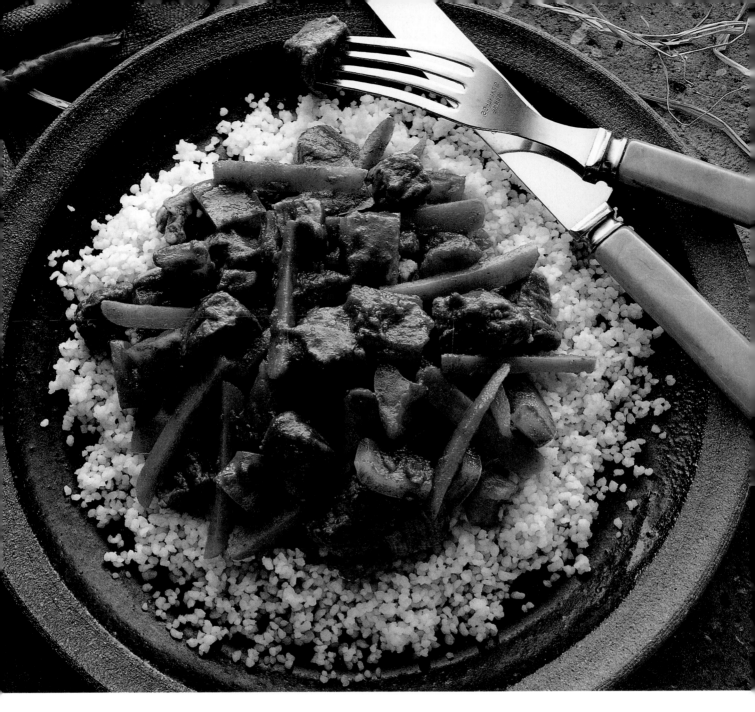

Ragout of Lamb

1- lb. well-trimmed
    boneless lamb leg roast,
    cut into 1/2-inch pieces
1 1/2 cups carrot strips
    (1 1/2 × 1/4-inch strips)
  2 teaspoons chili powder
1/2 teaspoon ground cinnamon
1/2 teaspoon sugar
1/4 teaspoon salt
  1 can (14 1/2 oz.) diced
    tomatoes
  1 cup green pepper chunks
    (1/2-inch chunks)

                4 servings

Place lamb pieces in 3-quart casserole. Cover. Microwave at High for 6 to 8 minutes, or just until meat is only slightly pink, stirring once or twice. Drain. Add remaining ingredients, except pepper chunks. Re-cover. Microwave at High for 5 minutes. Stir in pepper chunks. Re-cover. Microwave at High for 8 to 11 minutes, or until vegetables are tender, stirring twice.

Serving suggestion: Serve over hot cooked couscous or rice.

Per Serving: Calories: 214 • Protein: 26 g. • Carbohydrate: 11 g. • Fat: 7 g.
• Cholesterol: 76 mg. • Sodium: 388 mg.
Exchanges: 3 lean meat, 2 vegetable

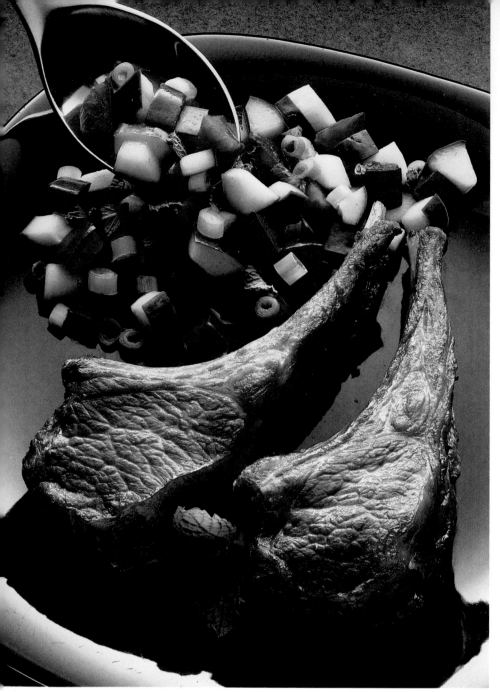

Lamb Chops & Mint Salsa

- ½ cup sliced green onions
- 1 clove garlic, minced
- 1 cup seeded chopped cucumber
- 1 medium tomato, seeded and chopped
- ¼ cup snipped fresh mint leaves
- ¼ teaspoon salt
- 8 well-trimmed lamb rib or loin chops (approx. 6 oz. each), 1 inch thick

4 servings

In 1-quart casserole, combine onions and garlic. Cover. Microwave at High for 2 to 3 minutes, or until onions are tender, stirring once. Add remaining ingredients, except chops. Mix well. Set salsa aside. Arrange chops on rack in broiler pan. Place under conventional broiler, with surface of meat 3 to 4 inches from heat. Broil for 7 to 11 minutes, or until desired doneness, turning chops over once. Serve with salsa.

Serving suggestion: Serve with warm pita bread.

Per Serving: Calories: 231 • Protein: 26 g.
• Carbohydrate: 4 g. • Fat: 12 g.
• Cholesterol: 83 mg. • Sodium: 217 mg.
Exchanges: 3 lean meat, 1 vegetable,
½ fat

Veal Florentine

- 1- lb. well-trimmed boneless veal leg rump roast or boneless veal shoulder roast, cut into 1-inch cubes
- ¾ cup diced carrot
- 2 tablespoons margarine or butter
- ¼ cup all-purpose flour
- 1 teaspoon salt
- ½ teaspoon pepper
- 2 cups skim milk
- 2 cups torn fresh spinach leaves

4 servings

Spray 12-inch nonstick skillet with nonstick vegetable cooking spray. Heat skillet conventionally over medium-high heat. Cook veal cubes for 6 to 8 minutes, or just until meat is no longer pink, stirring occasionally. Cover to keep warm. Set aside. In 2-quart casserole, combine carrot and margarine. Cover. Microwave at High for 3 to 4 minutes, or until carrot is tender-crisp, stirring once. Stir in flour, salt and pepper. Blend in milk. Microwave at High, uncovered, for 10 to 12 minutes, or until mixture thickens and bubbles, stirring 2 or 3 times. Add spinach and veal. Mix well.

Serving suggestion: Serve over hot cooked fettucini and garnish with freshly grated nutmeg.

Per Serving: Calories: 265 • Protein: 29 g. • Carbohydrate: 15 g. • Fat: 9 g.
• Cholesterol: 92 mg. • Sodium: 801 mg.
Exchanges: ¼ starch, 3 lean meat, 1 vegetable, ½ skim milk

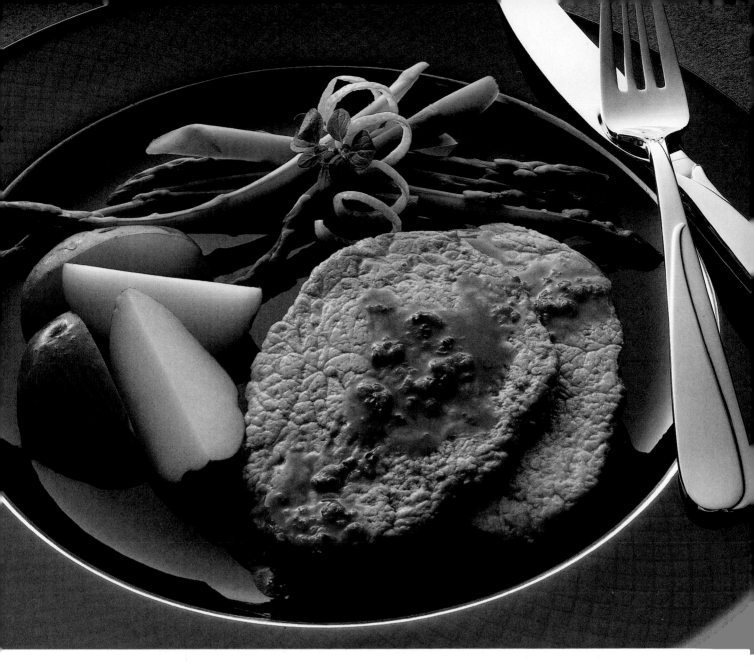

Lemon Veal & Asparagus

1 lb. fresh asparagus spears, trimmed and sliced in half lengthwise
1 tablespoon olive oil
1 teaspoon grated lemon peel, divided
½ teaspoon dried marjoram leaves, divided
1 lb. veal leg cutlets, ¼ inch thick (about 8 pieces)
⅛ teaspoon white pepper
½ cup dry white wine
1 teaspoon margarine or butter

4 servings

Place asparagus in 8-inch square baking dish. Sprinkle with oil, ½ teaspoon peel and ¼ teaspoon marjoram. Cover with plastic wrap. Microwave at High for 4 to 5 minutes, or until asparagus is tender-crisp, rearranging spears once. Cover to keep warm. Set aside. Sprinkle veal cutlets evenly with white pepper. Spray 12-inch non-stick skillet with nonstick vegetable cooking spray. Heat skillet conventionally over medium-high heat. Cook veal for 2 to 4 minutes, or just until meat is no longer pink. Remove from skillet. Cover to keep warm. Set aside. Add wine to skillet. Cook over medium-high heat for 1 to 2 minutes, or until reduced by half, stirring constantly. Stir in margarine, remaining ½ teaspoon peel and ¼ teaspoon marjoram. Remove from heat. Arrange veal cutlets and asparagus on serving platter. Spoon sauce over veal.

Serving suggestion: Serve with steamed new potatoes.

Per Serving: Calories: 196 • Protein: 26 g. • Carbohydrate: 3 g. • Fat: 7 g.
• Cholesterol: 89 mg. • Sodium: 87 mg.
Exchanges: 3 lean meat, ¾ vegetable

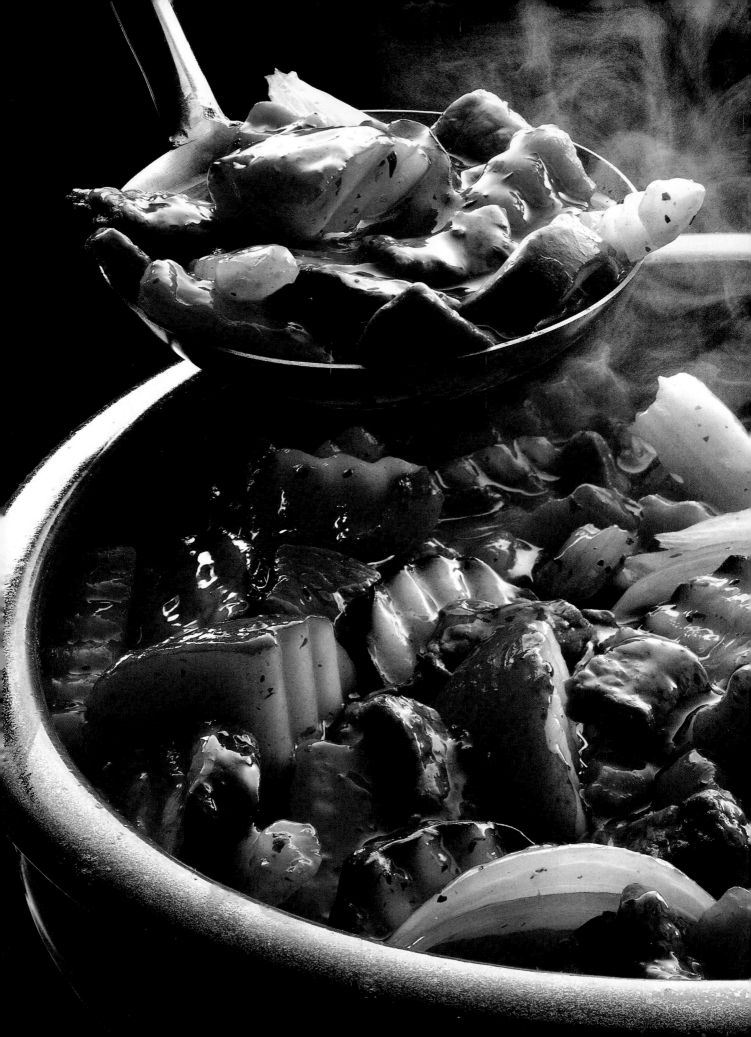

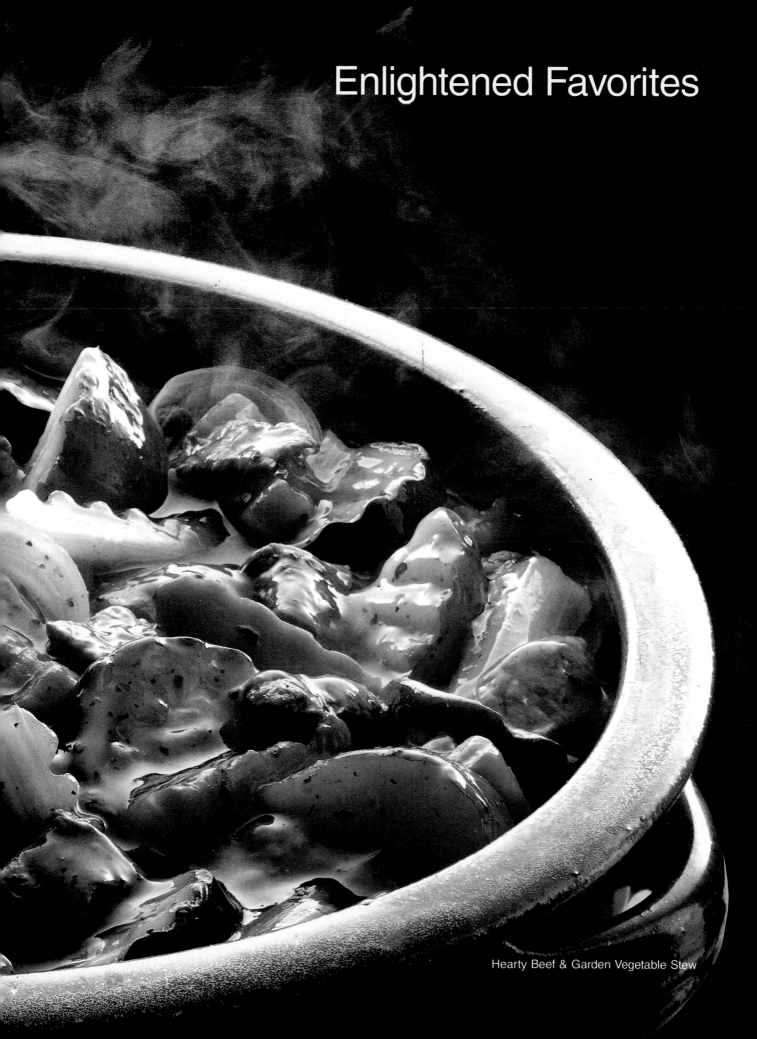

Enlightened Favorites

Hearty Beef & Garden Vegetable Stew

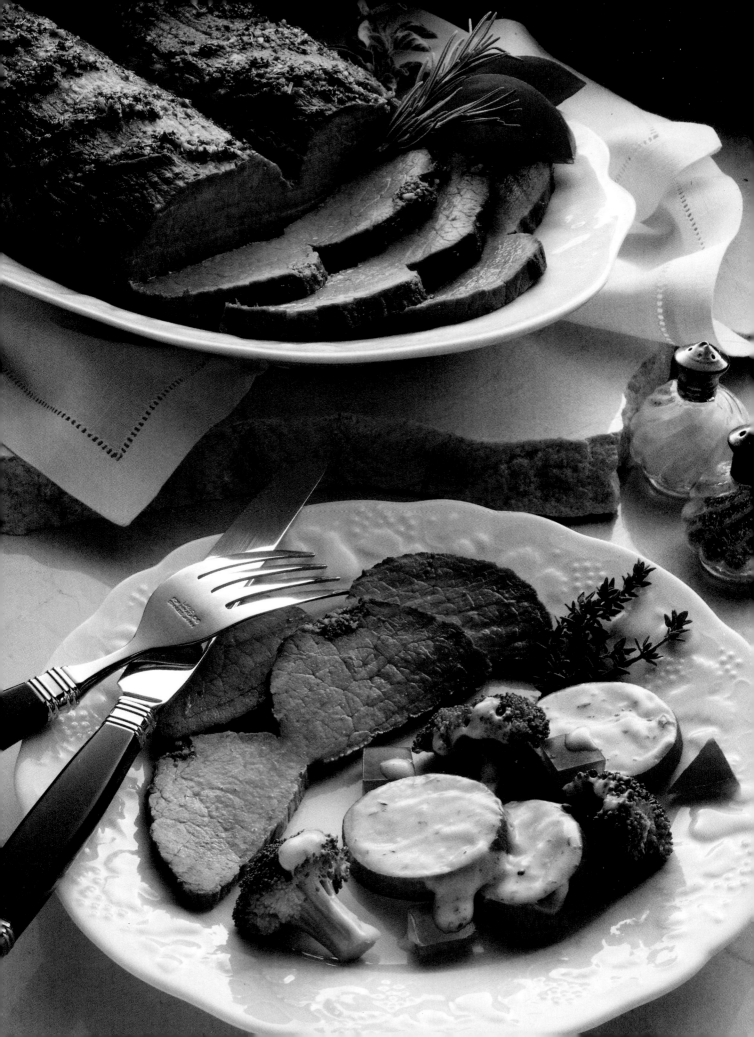

Beef

◄ Butterflied Eye Round Roast Italiano

1 tablespoon minced fresh garlic
2 teaspoons Italian seasoning
1/4 teaspoon freshly ground pepper
1 teaspoon olive oil
3 1/2 to 4-lb. beef eye round roast

14 to 16 servings

In small bowl, combine garlic, Italian seasoning, pepper and oil. Set seasoning mixture aside.

To butterfly roast, make horizontal cut through center of roast to within 1/2 inch of opposite side; do not cut through. Open roast like a book. Using tip of knife, cut 3/4-inch slits randomly over top surface of roast. Stuff seasoning mixture evenly into slits. Place roast in large plastic food-storage bag. Secure bag. Refrigerate 8 hours or overnight.

Remove roast from bag. Place roast, slit-side-up, on rack in broiler pan. Broil roast conventionally, with surface of meat 5 to 7 inches from heat, for 20 to 30 minutes for rare (135°F) to medium (155°F), or to desired doneness, rotating pan 2 or 3 times. Let roast stand, tented with foil, for 10 minutes before carving. (Internal temperature will rise 5°F during standing.) Carve roast across grain into thin slices.

Serving suggestions: Serve with Italian Scalloped Potatoes, right. Serve leftover Butterflied Eye Round Roast Italiano thinly sliced for sandwiches or use in Italian Roast Beef Hash, page 92.

Note: Tightly wrap and refrigerate any leftover beef up to 4 days, or package in freezer containers or bags and freeze 3 months.

Per Serving: Calories: 147 • Protein: 25 g. • Carbohydrate: 0 • Fat: 4 g. • Cholesterol: 59 mg. • Sodium: 55 mg.
Exchanges: 3 lean meat

◄ Italian Scalloped Potatoes

3 medium red potatoes, cut into 1/4-inch slices (about 1 lb.)
1/2 cup water, divided
8 oz. fresh broccoli flowerets
1/2 cup seeded chopped tomato
1 tablespoon margarine or butter
1 tablespoon all-purpose flour
1/2 teaspoon Italian seasoning
1/4 teaspoon salt
2/3 cup 2% milk

6 servings

In 2-quart casserole, combine potatoes and 1/4 cup water. Cover. Microwave at High for 6 to 10 minutes, or until tender, stirring once. Drain. Remove potatoes from casserole. Set aside.

In same casserole, combine broccoli and remaining 1/4 cup water. Cover. Microwave at High for 3 to 5 minutes, or until broccoli is very hot and color brightens. Drain.

In 1 1/2-quart microwave-safe gratin dish or 9-inch round cake dish, arrange potato slices and broccoli flowerets in alternating rows. Sprinkle with tomato. Set aside.

In 4-cup measure, microwave margarine at High for 45 seconds to 1 minute, or until melted. Stir in flour, Italian seasoning and salt. Blend in milk. Microwave at High for 2 1/2 to 5 1/2 minutes, or until mixture thickens and bubbles. Pour evenly over vegetables. Cover with plastic wrap. Microwave at High for 2 to 3 minutes, or until hot, rotating once.

Serving suggestion: Serve with Butterflied Eye Round Roast Italiano, left.

Per Serving: Calories: 104 • Protein: 4 g. • Carbohydrate: 17 g. • Fat: 3 g. • Cholesterol: 2 mg. • Sodium: 142 mg.
Exchanges: 2/3 starch, 1 vegetable, 1/2 fat

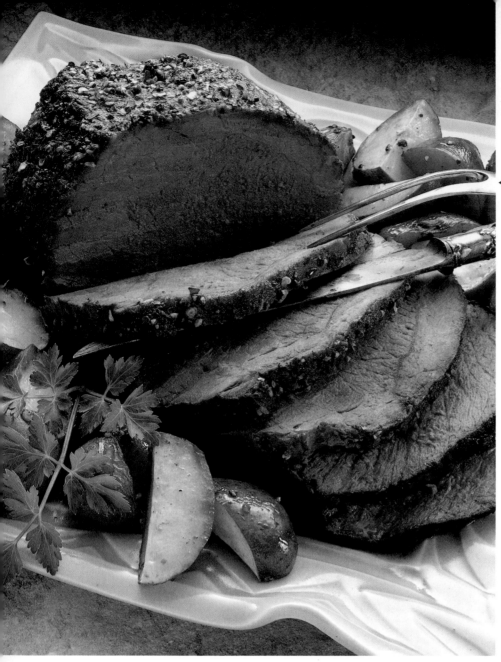

◄ Sirloin Roast au Poivre

◄ Sirloin Roast au Poivre

- 1 teaspoon whole black peppercorns
- 1 teaspoon whole green peppercorns
- 1 teaspoon whole white peppercorns
- 1 teaspoon paprika
- ¼ teaspoon crushed red pepper flakes
- 2½ to 3-lb. beef round tip roast (sirloin tip roast)

10 to 12 servings

In heavy-duty plastic bag, combine peppercorns. Remove air from bag and secure. Place on flat surface. Pound peppercorns with rolling pin to coarsely crush. Pour crushed peppercorns into small bowl. Add paprika and crushed red pepper flakes. Mix well. Place roast on rack in roasting pan. Pat peppercorn mixture evenly over exterior of roast, pressing firmly.

Insert meat thermometer. Roast conventionally for 1 hour 30 minutes to 1 hour 50 minutes for medium-rare (145°F) to medium (155°F), or to desired doneness. Let roast stand, tented with foil, for 10 minutes. (Internal temperature will rise 5°F during standing.) Carve roast across grain into thin slices.

Serving suggestion: Serve with Golden Roasted Potatoes, left, or chill and serve thinly sliced for sandwiches.

Note: Tightly wrap and refrigerate any leftover beef up to 4 days, or package in freezer containers or bags and freeze 3 months.

Per Serving: Calories: 160 • Protein: 25 g.
• Carbohydrate: 1 g. • Fat: 6 g.
• Cholesterol: 69 mg. • Sodium: 56 mg.
Exchanges: 3 lean meat

Golden Roasted Potatoes ▲

- 16 small new potatoes, cut into quarters (about 1½ lbs.)
- ½ cup water
- ½ cup condensed beef broth
- ¼ teaspoon garlic powder
  Snipped fresh parsley

4 to 6 servings

Heat conventional oven to 325°F. Place potatoes and water in 2-quart casserole. Cover. Microwave at High for 13 to 15 minutes, or until potatoes are tender, stirring 2 or 3 times. Drain. Set aside.

Place broth and garlic powder in 10 × 6-inch baking pan. Add potatoes. Stir to coat potatoes with broth mixture. Bake conventionally for 30 to 45 minutes, or until potatoes are golden brown and hot, stirring 3 or 4 times. Before serving, sprinkle with parsley.

Serving suggestion: Serve with Sirloin Roast au Poivre, right.

Per Serving: Calories: 136 • Protein: 4 g. • Carbohydrate: 30 g. • Fat: 0
• Cholesterol: 0 • Sodium: 177 mg.
Exchanges: 2 starch

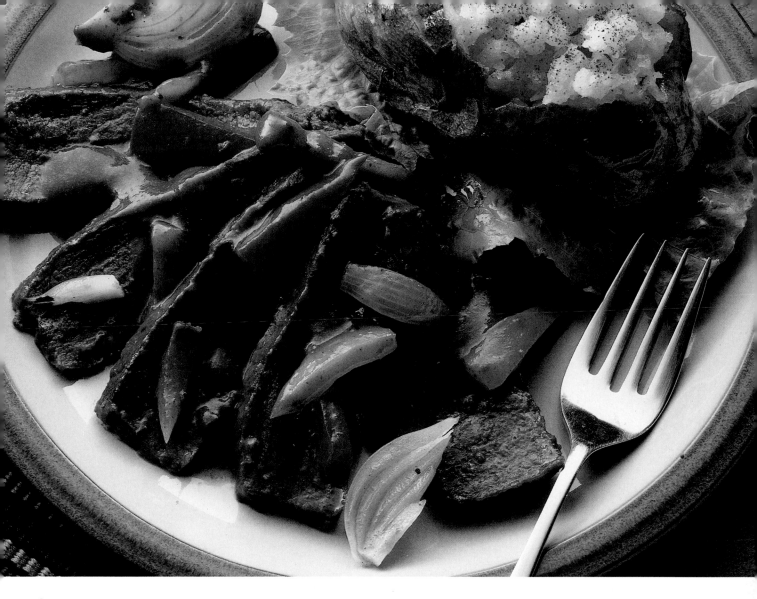

Southwestern-style Pot Roast

Sauce:

1 can (8 oz.) tomato sauce
¼ cup red wine vinegar
2 tablespoons tomato paste
2 tablespoons all-purpose flour
2 teaspoons sugar
2 teaspoons dried oregano leaves
1 teaspoon ground cumin
½ teaspoon ground cinnamon
½ teaspoon salt
½ teaspoon freshly ground pepper

3- lb. well-trimmed bone-in beef chuck
    arm pot roast, 1 ½ inches thick
3 jalapeño peppers, seeded and cut into
    ⅛-inch strips
1 medium onion, cut into 8 wedges
1 green pepper, cut into ½-inch strips
½ red pepper, cut into ½-inch strips
½ yellow pepper, cut into ½-inch strips

6 servings

In 2-cup measure, combine all sauce ingredients. Place roast in 10-inch square casserole. Pour sauce over meat. Sprinkle jalapeño strips over sauce. Arrange onion around meat. Cover. Microwave at High for 5 minutes. Microwave at 50% (Medium) for 45 minutes longer, rotating casserole once. Turn meat over. Microwave at 50% (Medium) for 35 to 45 minutes, or until meat is tender, rotating casserole and spooning sauce over meat once.

Add pepper strips. Re-cover. Microwave at 50% (Medium) for 8 to 10 minutes, or until pepper strips are tender-crisp. Let stand, covered, for 10 minutes. Carve meat across grain into thin slices and top with sauce and peppers. Serve extra sauce separately.

Serving suggestion: Serve with baked potato or hot cooked rice.

Per Serving: Calories: 259 • Protein: 35 g. • Carbohydrate: 13 g. • Fat: 7 g. • Cholesterol: 93 mg. • Sodium: 561 mg. Exchanges: ¼ starch, 4 lean meat, 2 vegetable

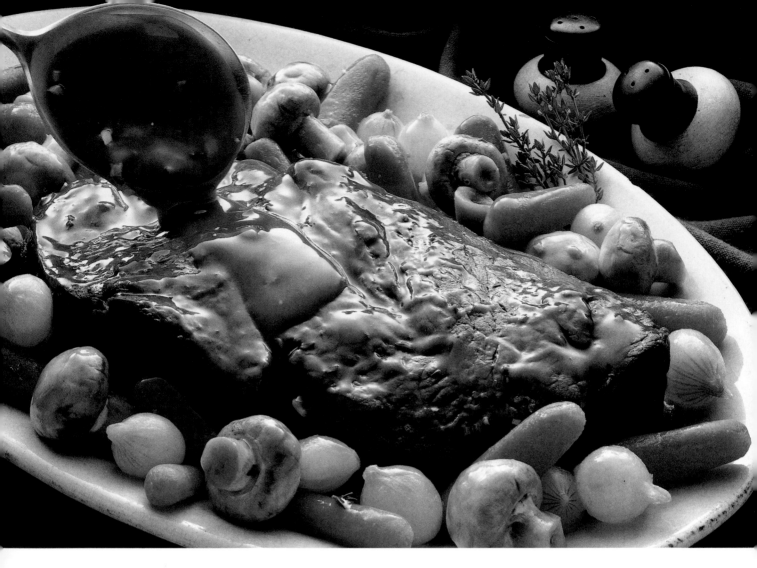

Burgundy Roast

3 tablespoons all-purpose
  flour, divided
2 teaspoons instant beef
  bouillon granules
1 teaspoon chopped fresh
  thyme leaves or
  1/2 teaspoon dried thyme
  leaves
2 cloves garlic, minced
1/4 teaspoon salt
1/3 cup Burgundy or other dry
  red wine
1/4 cup water
2- lb. well-trimmed boneless
  beef chuck shoulder roast,
  1 1/2 inches thick
8 oz. fresh mushrooms, stems
  trimmed (2 cups)
1 cup frozen pearl onions
1 cup frozen whole baby
  carrots

6 servings

In 1-cup measure, combine 2 tablespoons flour, the bouillon, thyme, garlic and salt. Blend in wine and water. Set aside.

Place remaining 1 tablespoon flour in large oven cooking bag. Hold bag closed at top and shake to coat. Place bag in 10-inch square casserole. Add roast to bag. Pour wine mixture over meat. Secure bag with nylon tie. Make six 1/2-inch slits in neck of bag below tie.

Microwave at High for 5 minutes. Microwave at 50% (Medium) for 25 minutes longer, rotating casserole once. Turn meat over. Add vegetables to bag. Secure bag. Microwave at 50% (Medium) for 25 to 35 minutes, or until meat is tender, rotating casserole once. Let bag stand, closed, for 10 minutes.

Serving suggestion: Serve with hot cooked wide egg noodles or rice.

Per Serving: Calories: 187 • Protein: 24 g. • Carbohydrate: 11 g. • Fat: 5 g.
• Cholesterol: 62 mg. • Sodium: 461 mg.
Exchanges: 3 lean meat, 1 vegetable, 1/3 fruit

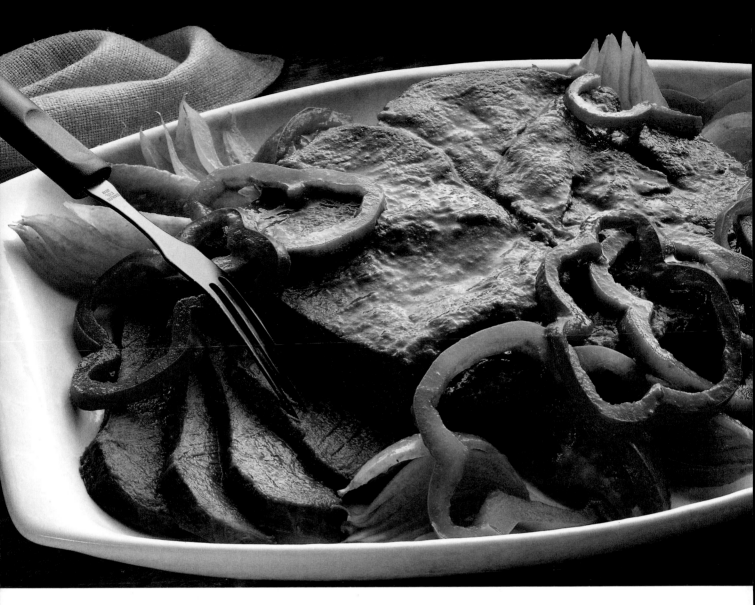

Pepper Steak Pot Roast

1 tablespoon cornstarch
1¼-lb. well-trimmed
   boneless beef chuck arm
   pot roast, 1½ inches thick
1 medium onion, cut into
   6 wedges
1 can (8 oz.) tomato sauce
2 tablespoons reduced-
   sodium soy sauce
1 teaspoon grated fresh
   gingerroot
2 cloves garlic, minced
1 teaspoon sugar
1 medium red pepper, cut
   into ¼-inch rings
1 medium green pepper, cut
   into ¼-inch rings
1 medium tomato, cut into
   6 wedges

4 servings

Place cornstarch in large oven cooking bag. Hold bag closed at top and shake to coat. Add roast and onion to bag. Set aside.

In medium mixing bowl, combine tomato sauce, soy sauce, ginger-root, garlic and sugar. Add to bag. Secure bag with nylon tie. Place in 10-inch square casserole. Make six ½-inch slits in neck of bag below tie.

Microwave at High for 5 minutes. Microwave at 50% (Medium) for 40 minutes longer, rotating casserole once. Add pepper rings and tomato to bag. Secure bag with nylon tie. Microwave at 50% (Medium) for 10 to 25 minutes, or until meat is tender, rotating casserole once. Let bag stand, closed, for 10 minutes.

Serving suggestion: Serve with hot cooked rice or baked potatoes.

Per Serving: Calories: 270 • Protein: 33 g. • Carbohydrate: 19 g. • Fat: 7 g.
• Cholesterol: 85 mg. • Sodium: 746 mg.
Exchanges: 3 lean meat, 4 vegetable

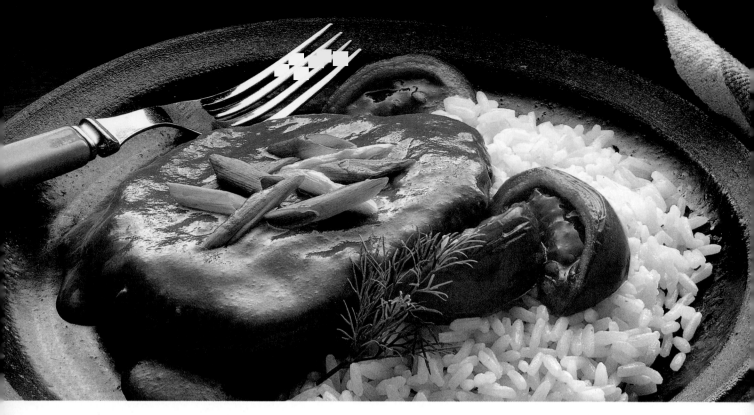

Tomato-Dill Steak Suisse ▲

1 - lb. well-trimmed beef top
   round steak, 1/2 to 3/4 inch
   thick, cut into 4 serving-
   size pieces
3 tablespoons all-purpose
   flour
1/2 teaspoon dry mustard
1/4 teaspoon freshly ground
   pepper
1 tablespoon vegetable oil
1 can (8 oz.) tomato sauce
2/3 cup water

2 medium tomatoes, each
   cut into 8 wedges, divided
1 teaspoon instant beef
   bouillon granules
1/2 teaspoon dill seed
1 bay leaf
1/4 teaspoon instant minced
   garlic
4 green onions, sliced
   diagonally into 1-inch
   lengths (1/2 cup)

4 servings

Pound beef pieces to 1/4-inch thickness. Set aside. In large plastic food-storage bag, combine flour, mustard and pepper. In 12-inch nonstick skillet, heat oil conventionally over medium-high heat. Add meat, one piece at a time, to flour mixture. Shake to coat. Reserve any remaining flour mixture. Add meat to skillet. Cook for 4 to 5 minutes, or just until meat is browned on both sides. Arrange in single layer in 10-inch square casserole. Set aside.

In medium mixing bowl, combine tomato sauce, water, half of tomato wedges, the bouillon, dill seed, bay leaf, garlic and remaining flour mixture. Pour over meat in casserole. Cover. Microwave at High for 5 minutes. Microwave at 50% (Medium) for 40 to 45 minutes longer, or until meat is tender, adding remaining tomato wedges and onions during last 5 minutes of cooking time. Before serving, let stand, covered, for 10 minutes.

Serving suggestion: Serve with hot cooked rice.

Per Serving: Calories: 308 • Protein: 32 g. • Carbohydrate: 15 g. • Fat: 14 g.
• Cholesterol: 77 mg. • Sodium: 601 mg.
Exchanges: 1/4 starch, 3 lean meat, 2 vegetable, 3/4 fat

Cranberry-Orange Barbecue Beef

1 can (8 oz.) tomato sauce
1/2 cup frozen cranberry-orange
   sauce, defrosted
1 tablespoon packed brown
   sugar
2 teaspoons chili powder
1 teaspoon Dijon mustard
1/4 teaspoon salt
1 - lb. beef round tip steak
   (sirloin tip roast), cut into
   2 × 3/4 × 1/4-inch-thick strips

4 servings

In 2-quart casserole, combine all ingredients, except beef strips. Stir in meat. Mix well. Cover. Microwave at High for 3 minutes. Stir. Microwave at 50% (Medium) for 40 to 50 minutes longer, or until meat is tender, stirring 2 or 3 times.

Serving suggestion: Serve meat mixture over hot cooked rice or split kaiser rolls.

Per Serving: Calories: 237 • Protein: 25 g.
• Carbohydrate: 24 g. • Fat: 5 g.
• Cholesterol: 68 mg. • Sodium: 611 mg.
Exchanges: 3 lean meat, 1/2 vegetable,
1 1/2 fruit

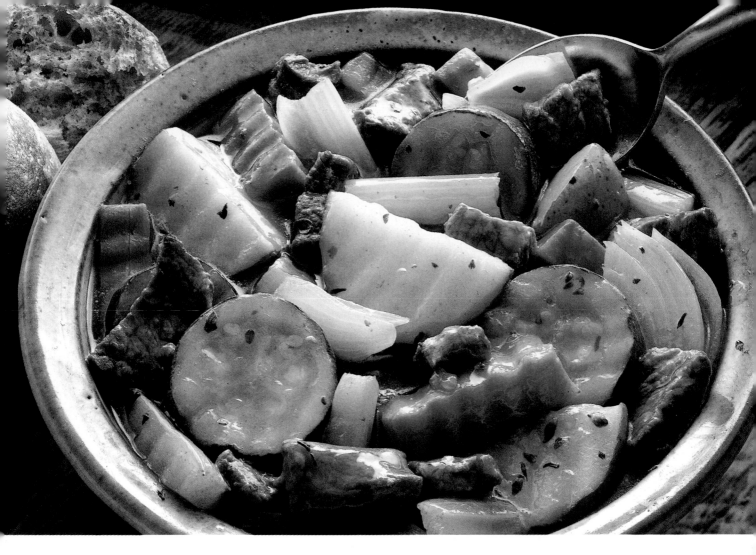

Hearty Beef & Garden Vegetable Stew

1- lb. well-trimmed beef top round steak,
    1/2 to 3/4 inch thick, cut across grain into
    1 × 1/4-inch-thick strips
4 to 6 small new potatoes, crinkle-cut into
    quarters (about 1/2 lb.)
1 1/2 cups crinkle-cut carrot chunks (1 1/2 × 1/2-inch
    chunks)
2 medium zucchini, crinkle-cut into 1/2-inch
    slices
1 stalk celery, crinkle-cut into 1 1/2 × 1/2-inch
    chunks
1 medium onion, cut into 8 wedges
2 cups ready-to-serve beef broth, divided
1 teaspoon dried thyme leaves
1 teaspoon dried marjoram leaves
1/2 teaspoon salt
1/8 teaspoon freshly ground pepper
2 tablespoons plus 1 teaspoon cornstarch

4 servings

Place beef strips in 2-quart casserole. Cover. Microwave at High for 5 to 7 minutes, or just until meat is no longer pink, stirring once. Drain. Cover to keep warm. Set aside.

Place vegetables in 10-inch square casserole. Set aside. In 1-cup measure, combine 1 cup broth, the thyme, marjoram, salt and pepper. Pour over vegetables. Cover. Microwave at High for 15 to 26 minutes, or until potatoes are tender, stirring twice. Add meat to vegetables. Cover to keep warm. Set aside.

In 2-cup measure, combine remaining 1 cup broth and the cornstarch. Microwave at High for 3 to 5 minutes, or until sauce is thickened and translucent, stirring once or twice. Pour sauce over vegetable mixture. Mix well. Microwave at High, uncovered, for 2 to 3 minutes, or until mixture is hot, stirring once.

Serving suggestion: Serve with whole-grain bread or soft bread sticks.

Per Serving: Calories: 301 • Protein: 31 g. • Carbohydrate: 26 g.
• Fat: 8 g. • Cholesterol: 82 mg. • Sodium: 761 mg.
Exchanges: 3/4 starch, 3 lean meat, 3 vegetable

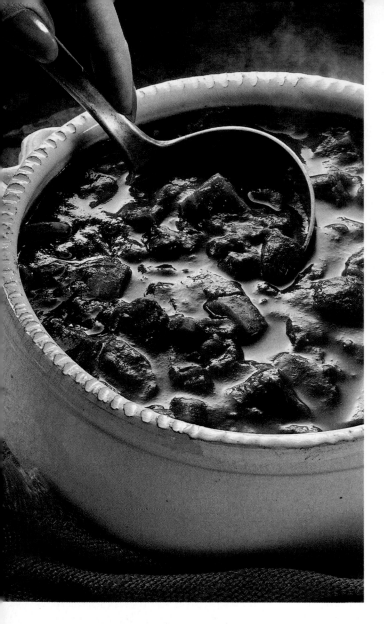

Authentic Texas-style Chili con Carne

- 1 cup chopped onions
- 1 cup chopped green pepper
- 2 cloves garlic, minced
- 2 teaspoons olive oil
- 1 can (28 oz.) whole tomatoes, undrained and cut up
- 1 can (8 oz.) tomato sauce
- 1 can (4 oz.) chopped green chilies
- ¼ cup plus 2 tablespoons tomato paste
- 1 to 2 tablespoons diced canned jalapeño peppers (optional)
- 1 tablespoon plus 1 teaspoon chili powder
- 2 teaspoons cocoa
- 1½ teaspoons dried oregano leaves
- 1½ teaspoons ground cumin
- ½ teaspoon ground cinnamon
- ½ teaspoon salt
- ½ teaspoon freshly ground pepper
- 1-lb. beef round tip steak, cut into 1 × ½ × ¼-inch-thick strips*
- ½ cup shredded reduced-fat Cheddar cheese (5 g. fat per oz.)
- ¼ cup light sour cream

4 servings

Serving suggestion: Serve with corn bread sticks or muffins.

*Substitute 1-lb. well-trimmed boneless beef bottom round steak, ½ to ¾ inch thick, for round tip steak.

Per Serving: Calories: 372 • Protein: 35 g. • Carbohydrate: 28 g. • Fat: 15 g. • Cholesterol: 84 mg. • Sodium: 1491 mg. Exchanges: 3½ starch, 5 vegetable, 1 fat

How to Make Authentic Texas-style Chili con Carne

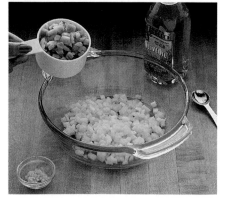

Combine onions, green pepper, garlic and oil in 3-quart casserole. Cover. Microwave at High for 6 to 8 minutes, or until onions are tender. Add remaining ingredients, except beef strips, cheese and sour cream. Mix well. Cover. Set aside.

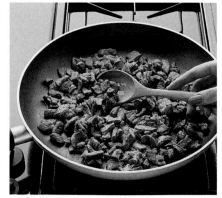

Spray 12-inch nonstick skillet with nonstick vegetable cooking spray. Heat skillet conventionally over medium-high heat. Add beef strips. Cook for 5 to 7 minutes, or just until meat is slightly browned and no longer pink, turning over once. Drain.

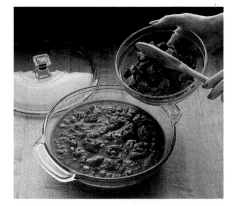

Add meat to chili mixture. Mix well. Re-cover. Microwave at High for 5 minutes. Microwave at 50% (Medium) for 1 hour to 1 hour 15 minutes longer, or until meat is tender, stirring 3 or 4 times. Divide chili evenly among 4 bowls. Top each serving evenly with cheese and sour cream.

Chunky Beef & Spaghetti Soup

     1 jar (14 oz.) spaghetti sauce
2 1/2 cups hot water
    1/2 cup chopped onion
    1/2 cup broken uncooked
        spaghetti
     6 oz. fresh mushrooms, sliced
        (1 1/2 cups)
    1/2 cup thinly sliced green
        pepper
     1 medium tomato, seeded
        and chopped
     1 small zucchini, thinly sliced
  1- lb. well-trimmed beef
        top round steak, 1/2 to
        3/4 inch thick, cut across
        grain into 1 × 1/4-inch-thick
        strips
     1 teaspoon Italian seasoning
    1/4 teaspoon garlic powder

4 servings

In 2-quart casserole, combine spaghetti sauce, water, onion and spaghetti. Cover. Microwave at High for 15 to 20 minutes, or just until spaghetti is tender, stirring 2 or 3 times. Add mushrooms, green pepper, tomato and zucchini. Mix well. Re-cover. Microwave at High for 5 to 8 minutes, or until vegetables are tender-crisp and mixture is hot, stirring once. Cover to keep warm. Set soup aside.

Place beef strips in 2-quart casserole. Sprinkle with Italian seasoning and garlic powder. Mix well. Cover. Microwave at High for 4 to 5 minutes, or just until meat is only slightly pink, stirring once or twice. Drain. Add meat to soup. Mix well.

Serving suggestion: Sprinkle each serving with Parmesan cheese-flavored croutons.

Per Serving: Calories: 371 • Protein: 36 g.
• Carbohydrate: 34 g. • Fat: 10 g.
• Cholesterol: 77 mg. • Sodium: 543 mg.
Exchanges: 2 starch, 3 1/2 lean meat,
1 vegetable

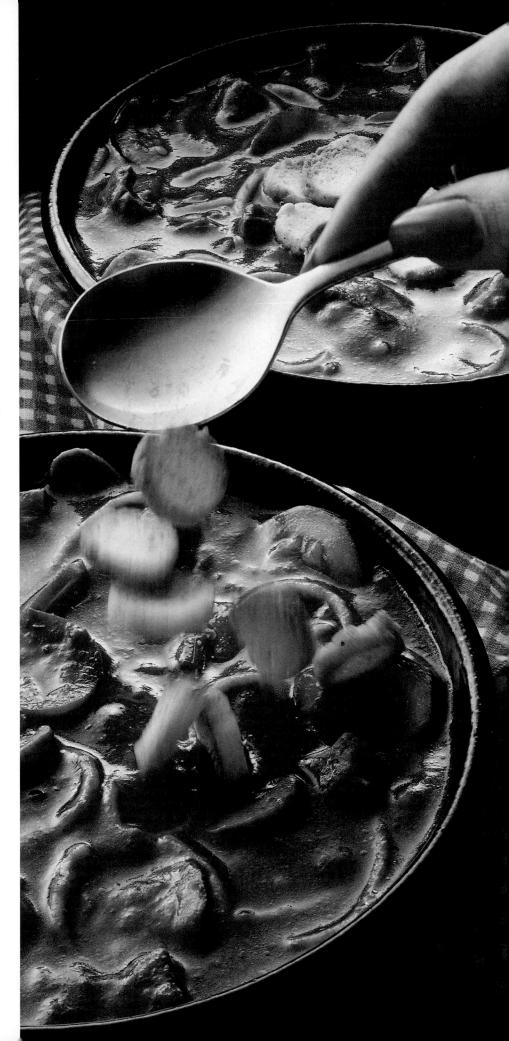

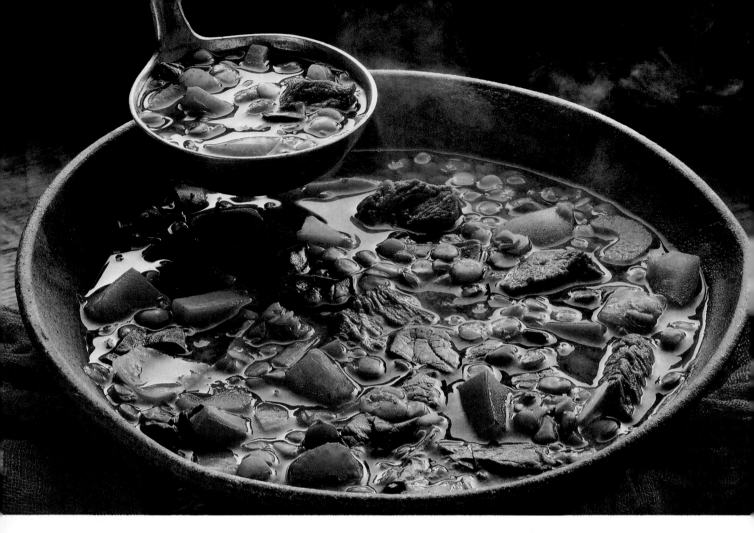

Lentil Beef & Spinach Stew

    1 cup chopped onions
    1 stalk celery, chopped
       (¾ cup)
    2 cloves garlic, minced
    1 tablespoon plus 1 teaspoon
       olive oil, divided
    2 cups hot water
    1 can (14½ oz.) ready-to-
       serve beef broth
 1¼   cups dried lentils (8 oz.)
    1 teaspoon dried thyme leaves
    ¾ teaspoon dried oregano
       leaves
    2 lbs. beef shank crosscuts,
       cut 1 inch thick
    1 cup carrot strips
       (1 × ¼-inch strips)
    4 cups chopped fresh
       spinach leaves
    1 tablespoon lemon juice
    ½ teaspoon salt
    ½ teaspoon pepper
    1 medium tomato, seeded
       and chopped

6 servings

In 3-quart casserole, combine onions, celery, garlic and 2 teaspoons oil. Cover. Microwave at High for 5 to 7 minutes, or until onions are tender, stirring once. Add water, broth, lentils, thyme and oregano. Cover. Set aside.

In 12-inch nonstick skillet, heat remaining 2 teaspoons oil conventionally over medium-high heat. Add beef shanks. Cook for 8 to 10 minutes, or just until meat is browned on both sides. Cut meat from bones. Add meat to casserole. Mix well. Cover.

Microwave at High for 5 minutes. Stir. Microwave at 50% (Medium) for 45 to 50 minutes longer, or until lentils are tender, stirring 2 or 3 times. Add carrots. Re-cover. Microwave at 50% (Medium) for 10 to 13 minutes, or until carrots and meat are tender, stirring once. Remove meat from casserole. Set aside.

Add spinach, lemon juice, salt and pepper to stew. Mix well. Let stand, covered, for 5 minutes, or until spinach is wilted. Carve meat into bite-size pieces. Return meat to stew. Stir in tomato.

Serving suggestion: Serve with slices of heavy whole-grain bread.

Per Serving: Calories: 336 • Protein: 36 g. • Carbohydrate: 31 g. • Fat: 8 g.
• Cholesterol: 40 mg. • Sodium: 553 mg.
Exchanges: 1½ starch, 4 lean meat, 1½ vegetable

Spicy Beef & Vegetable Gumbo

- 2 teaspoons vegetable oil
- 2 lbs. beef shank crosscuts, cut 1 inch thick
- 1 can (28 oz.) whole tomatoes, cut up and undrained
- 1 can (14½ oz.) ready-to-serve chicken broth
- 1 pkg. (10 oz.) frozen sliced okra
- 1 cup chopped green pepper
- 1 cup chopped onions
- ⅓ cup uncooked brown rice
- 1 teaspoon dried thyme leaves
- ½ teaspoon dried oregano leaves
- ½ teaspoon garlic powder
- ¼ teaspoon freshly ground pepper
- ¼ teaspoon crushed red pepper flakes

4 servings

In 10-inch nonstick skillet, heat oil conventionally over medium-high heat. Add beef shanks. Cook for 8 to 10 minutes, or just until meat is browned on both sides. Cut meat from bones. Place meat in 3-quart casserole. Add remaining ingredients. Mix well. Cover.

Microwave at High for 5 minutes. Stir. Microwave at 50% (Medium), covered, for 1 hour 10 minutes to 1 hour 45 minutes longer, or until meat and rice are tender, stirring once or twice. Let stand, covered, for 10 minutes. Remove meat from casserole. Carve meat into bite-size pieces. Return meat to gumbo.

Serving suggestion: Serve with tossed green salad and crusty French bread.

Per Serving: Calories: 368 • Protein: 39 g. • Carbohydrate: 30 g. • Fat: 10 g. • Cholesterol: 59 mg. • Sodium: 871 mg. Exchanges: ¾ starch, 4 lean meat, 3¾ vegetable

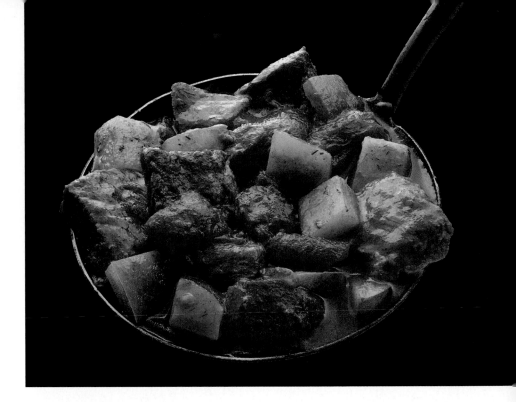

Hungarian Goulash ▲

- 1 cup chopped onions
- 1 teaspoon vegetable oil
- 1 can (28 oz.) whole tomatoes, undrained and cut up
- 1 lb. red potatoes, cut into ½-inch cubes (about 3 cups)
- 1 medium green pepper, cut into ½-inch chunks
- ¼ cup dry red wine
- 3 tablespoons tomato paste
- 1 tablespoon Hungarian paprika
- 1 teaspoon caraway seed
- 1 teaspoon dried dill weed
- 1 teaspoon sugar
- ½ teaspoon salt
- 1¼-lb. well-trimmed boneless beef chuck shoulder steak, 1 inch thick, cut into 1 × ¼-inch-thick strips
- ¼ cup light sour cream

4 servings

Place onions and oil in 3-quart casserole. Mix well. Cover. Microwave at High for 4 to 6 minutes, or until onions are tender-crisp, stirring once. Add remaining ingredients, except beef strips and sour cream. Mix well. Cover. Set aside.

Spray 12-inch nonstick skillet with nonstick vegetable cooking spray. Heat skillet conventionally over medium-high heat. Add beef strips. Cook for 5 to 7 minutes, or just until meat is no longer pink, turning over once. Drain.

Add meat to casserole. Mix well. Re-cover. Microwave at High for 5 minutes. Stir. Microwave at 50% (Medium) for 35 to 50 minutes longer, or until meat is tender, stirring 2 or 3 times. Divide goulash evenly among 4 bowls. Top each serving evenly with sour cream. Garnish with fresh dill sprigs, if desired.

Serving suggestion: Serve with crusty French bread or soft bread sticks.

Per Serving: Calories: 400 • Protein: 35 g. • Carbohydrate: 40 g. • Fat: 12 g. • Cholesterol: 91 mg. • Sodium: 763 mg. Exchanges: 1 starch, 3 lean meat, 5 vegetable, ½ fat

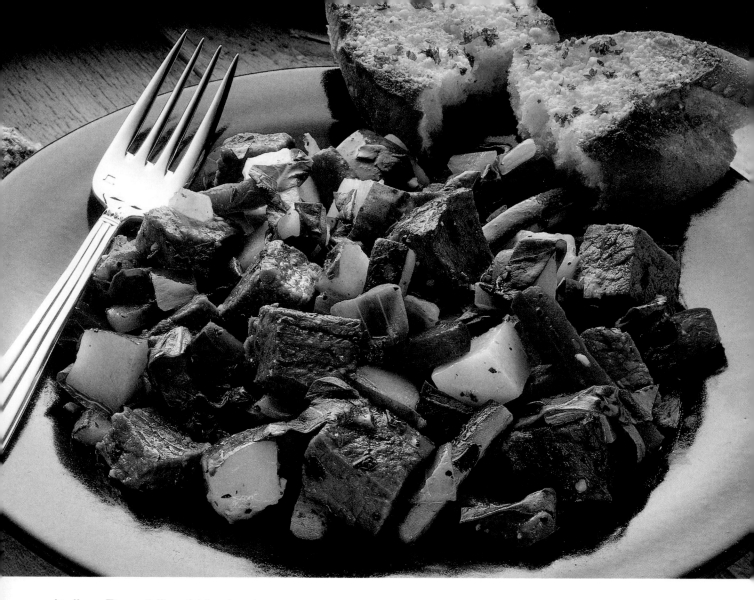

Italian Roast Beef Hash

1/2 cup chopped onion
1 clove garlic, minced
2 teaspoons olive oil
2 cups cubed red potatoes
    (1/2-inch cubes)
2 tablespoons water
1 cup zucchini strips
    (1 1/2 × 1/4-inch strips)
3/4 cup red pepper strips
    (1 1/2 × 1/4-inch strips)
1/2 teaspoon dried marjoram
    leaves
1/2 teaspoon dried basil leaves
1/4 to 1/2 teaspoon salt
1/4 teaspoon pepper
3/4 lb. leftover fully cooked
    roast beef, cut into 3/4-inch
    cubes*
1 cup chopped fresh spinach
    leaves

4 servings

In 2-quart casserole, combine onion, garlic and oil. Cover. Microwave at High for 4 to 5 minutes, or until onion is tender, stirring once. Add potatoes and water. Cover. Microwave at High for 8 to 10 minutes, or until potatoes are tender, stirring twice. Add remaining ingredients, except beef cubes and spinach. Mix well. Set aside.

Spray 12-inch nonstick skillet with nonstick vegetable cooking spray. Heat conventionally over medium-high heat. Add vegetable mixture. Cook for 2 to 4 minutes, or until zucchini is lightly browned, stirring frequently. Add meat and spinach. Cook for 1 1/2 to 2 minutes, or until meat is hot and spinach is wilted, stirring frequently.

Serving suggestion: Serve with toasted sourdough bread slices, sprinkled with grated fresh Parmesan cheese.

*Use leftovers from Butterflied Eye Round Roast Italiano, page 81, if desired.

Per Serving: Calories: 252 • Protein: 27 g. • Carbohydrate: 18 g. • Fat: 7 g.
• Cholesterol: 59 mg. • Sodium: 284 mg.
Exchanges: 3/4 starch, 3 lean meat, 1 1/2 vegetable

Chimichangas

2 tablespoons vegetable oil, divided
1 medium onion, thinly sliced
2 cloves garlic, minced
1 medium tomato, seeded and chopped
1 cup salsa
1 can (4 oz.) chopped green chilies, drained
1 teaspoon chili powder
1/2 teaspoon dried oregano leaves
3/4 lb. leftover fully cooked pot roast, shredded*
4 flour tortillas (10-inch) **

4 servings

Serving suggestion: Top with shredded reduced-fat cheese, light sour cream and seeded chopped tomato.

*Use leftover Southwestern-style Pot Roast, page 83, if desired.
**For easier rolling and less cracking, purchase "pressed" flour tortillas.

Per Serving: Calories: 366 • Protein: 29 g.
• Carbohydrate: 35 g. • Fat: 12 g.
• Cholesterol: 59 mg. • Sodium: 808 mg.
Exchanges: 2 starch, 3 lean meat,
1 vegetable, 1/2 fat

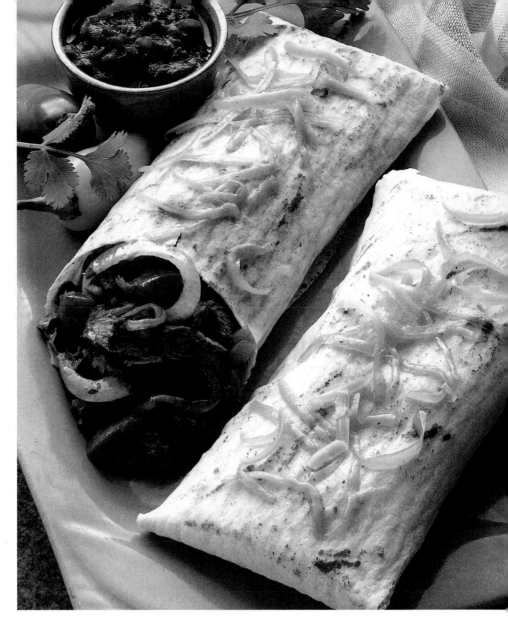

How to Make Chimichangas

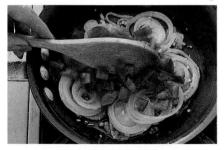

Heat 1 tablespoon oil conventionally in 12-inch nonstick skillet over medium-high heat. Add onion and garlic. Cook for 7 to 9 minutes, or until tender, stirring frequently. Reduce heat to medium. Add tomato, salsa, chilies, chili powder and oregano. Mix well.

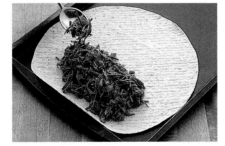

Stir in shredded beef. Cook for 10 to 12 minutes, or until mixture is slightly thickened and flavors are blended, stirring frequently. Heat conventional oven to 450°F. Brush large baking sheet lightly with some of remaining 1 tablespoon oil. Spoon one-fourth of meat mixture across bottom half of 1 tortilla, to within 1 1/2 inches of sides.

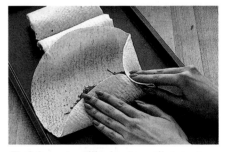

Fold up tortilla just until meat mixture is enclosed. Fold in sides. Roll up tortilla. Place seam-side-down on prepared baking sheet. Brush lightly with some of remaining oil. Repeat with remaining ingredients. Bake for 15 to 20 minutes, or until golden brown.

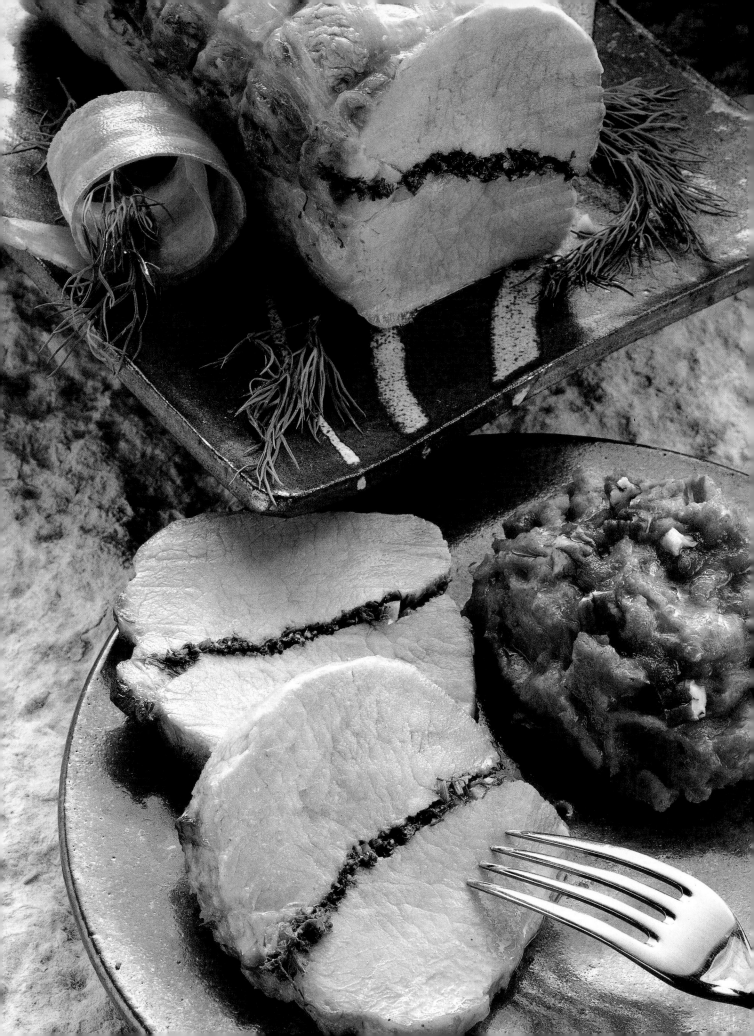

Pork

◄ Porketta

½ cup snipped fresh parsley
¼ cup snipped fresh dill weed
1 tablespoon minced fresh garlic
1 teaspoon fennel seed, crushed
½ teaspoon freshly ground pepper
¼ teaspoon salt
3½ to 4-lb. well-trimmed boneless pork
    double loin roast

14 to 16 servings

Heat conventional oven to 325°F. In medium mixing bowl, combine all ingredients, except roast. Set stuffing mixture aside.

Untie pork roast. Separate the two pieces of loin. Spoon and pack stuffing mixture on top of one pork loin piece. Place remaining loin piece over stuffing. Tie at 1½-inch intervals to secure. Place roast in 8-inch square baking dish. Cover with wax paper or microwave cooking paper. Microwave at 70% (Medium High) for 10 to 15 minutes, or just until exterior is no longer pink, turning roast over after half the cooking time.

Place roast on rack in roasting pan. Insert meat thermometer. Roast conventionally for 55 minutes to 1 hour 10 minutes, or until internal temperature registers 155°F and juices run clear. Let roast stand, tented with foil, for 10 minutes. (Internal temperature will rise 5°F during standing.) Carve roast across grain into thin slices.

Serving suggestion: Serve with Cinnamon-spiced Carrot & Potato Bake, right.

Note: Tightly wrap and refrigerate any leftover pork up to 4 days, or package in freezer containers or bags and freeze 3 to 4 months.

Per Serving: Calories: 170 • Protein: 24 g. • Carbohydrate: 1 g. • Fat: 8 g. • Cholesterol: 69 mg. • Sodium: 87 mg.
Exchanges: 3 lean meat

◄ Cinnamon-spiced Carrot & Potato Bake

1 lb. carrots, peeled and cut into 1-inch
    lengths
1 lb. russet potatoes, peeled and cut into
    1-inch chunks
¼ cup water
1 tablespoon packed brown sugar
1 tablespoon margarine or butter
½ teaspoon ground cinnamon
½ teaspoon salt
2 to 4 tablespoons milk

Topping:
1 tablespoon margarine or butter
1 tablespoon packed brown sugar
1 tablespoon chopped pecans

6 servings

Heat conventional oven to 325°F. In 2-quart casserole, combine carrots, potatoes and water. Cover. Microwave at High for 16 to 24 minutes, or until vegetables are very tender, stirring 2 or 3 times. Drain. Add 1 tablespoon sugar, 1 tablespoon margarine, the cinnamon and salt. Place mixture in food processor. Add 2 tablespoons milk. Process until mixture is smooth but stiff, adding additional milk, if necessary. Spoon mixture into 1-quart casserole or baking dish. Set aside.

In small mixing bowl, cut together topping ingredients until crumbly. Sprinkle over carrot and potato mixture. Bake conventionally for 15 to 25 minutes, or until topping is melted and mixture is hot.

Serving suggestion: Serve with Porketta, left.

Per Serving: Calories: 146 • Protein: 2 g. • Carbohydrate: 24 g. • Fat: 5 g. • Cholesterol: 1 mg. • Sodium: 260 mg.
Exchanges: ⅔ starch, 1 vegetable, ½ fruit, 1 fat

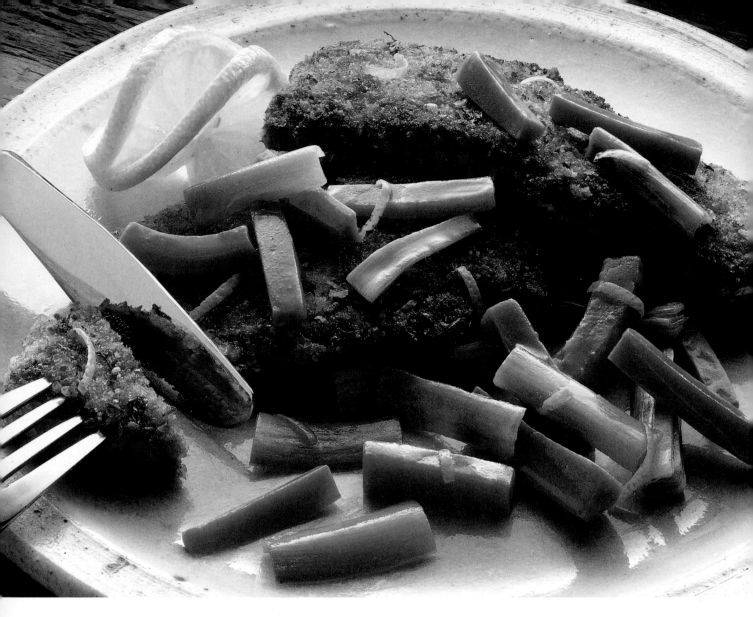

Lemony Pork Piccata

2 well-trimmed pork
    tenderloins (approx.
    1 lb. each), each cut
    crosswise into 6 pieces
1 cup unseasoned dry bread
    crumbs
1 tablespoon plus 1 teaspoon
    grated lemon peel, divided
1 tablespoon dried parsley
    flakes
2 or 3 egg whites
¼ cup olive oil, divided
1 cup carrot strips (2 × ¼-inch
    strips)
1 leek, cut in half lengthwise,
    rinsed and sliced crosswise
    (1-inch slices)
1 teaspoon margarine or
    butter

6 servings

Pound pork pieces lightly to ¼-inch thickness. Set aside.

In 1-quart casserole or shallow dish, combine bread crumbs, 1 table-spoon peel and the parsley. Place egg whites in another shallow dish. Dip 3 pork pieces first in egg white and then in crumb mixture, turning to coat both sides.

In 10-inch skillet, heat 1 tablespoon oil conventionally over medium heat. Add coated pork pieces. Cook for 3 to 5 minutes, or just until meat is no longer pink, turning over once. Place on serving platter. Cover to keep warm. Set aside. Wipe out skillet with paper towels. Repeat with remaining oil and pork.

In 1-quart casserole, combine carrot strips, leek and margarine. Cover. Microwave at High for 3 to 5 minutes, or until vegetables are tender, stirring once. Sprinkle with remaining 1 teaspoon peel. Toss to coat. Spoon mixture over pork.

Serving suggestion: Serve with hot cooked rice.

Per Serving: Calories: 385 • Protein: 39 g. • Carbohydrate: 19 g. • Fat: 18 g.
• Cholesterol: 108 mg. • Sodium: 240 mg.
Exchanges: 1 starch, 4 lean meat, 1 vegetable, 1¼ fat

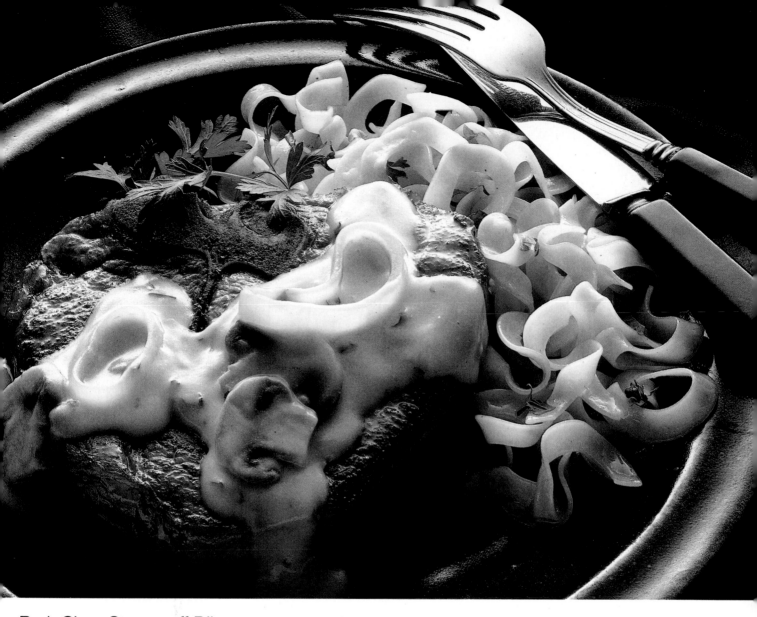

Pork Chop Stroganoff Dijon

8 oz. fresh mushrooms, sliced (2 cups)
1 cup sliced onions
1 tablespoon margarine or butter
2 tablespoons all-purpose flour
1 tablespoon Dijon mustard
1 tablespoon snipped fresh parsley
1/4 teaspoon freshly ground pepper
3/4 cup ready-to-serve chicken broth
4 well-trimmed bone-in pork center loin or rib chops (8 oz. each), 1 inch thick
2 tablespoons light sour cream

4 servings

In 8-inch square baking dish, combine mushrooms, onions and margarine. Cover with plastic wrap. Microwave at High for 3 1/2 to 5 minutes, or until vegetables are tender, stirring once. Stir in flour, mustard, parsley and pepper. Blend in broth. Set aside.

Spray 12-inch nonstick skillet with nonstick vegetable cooking spray. Heat conventionally over medium-high heat. Add pork chops. Cook for 5 to 6 minutes, or just until meat is browned on both sides. Arrange chops over mushroom mixture. Cover with plastic wrap. Microwave at 70% (Medium High) for 10 to 15 minutes, or just until meat is no longer pink, rotating dish twice and turning chops over once. Remove chops from baking dish. Place on serving platter. Cover to keep warm. Set aside.

Microwave mushroom mixture at High, uncovered, for 1 to 2 minutes, or until mixture thickens and bubbles, stirring once. Stir in sour cream. Spoon sauce over chops.

Serving suggestion: Serve with lightly buttered egg noodles.

Per Serving: Calories: 275 • Protein: 31 g. • Carbohydrate: 10 g. • Fat: 14 g.
• Cholesterol: 81 mg. • Sodium: 407 mg.
Exchanges: 3 lean meat, 2 vegetable, 1 fat

Far East Stroganoff ▶

¼ cup reduced-sodium
    teriyaki sauce
2 cloves garlic, minced
1 teaspoon ground ginger,
    divided
4 well-trimmed boneless pork
    sirloin chops (4 oz. each),
    ½ inch thick, cut into
    1 × ¼-inch-thick strips*
1 cup diagonally sliced
    carrots (⅛-inch slices)
1 tablespoon water
1 pkg. (6 oz.) frozen snow
    pea pods
8 oz. fresh mushrooms,
    sliced (2 cups)
¼ cup all-purpose flour
1 cup ready-to-serve beef
    broth
1 tablespoon reduced-sodium
    soy sauce
½ cup diagonally sliced
    green onions
½ cup light sour cream

4 servings

In medium mixing bowl, combine teriyaki sauce, garlic and ½ teaspoon ginger. Add pork strips. Mix well. Set aside.

Place carrots and water in 2-quart casserole. Cover. Microwave at High for 3 minutes. Add snow pea pods and mushrooms. Re-cover. Microwave at High for 5 to 7 minutes, or until carrots are tender-crisp, stirring once or twice. Drain. Set aside.

In 2-cup measure, combine flour and remaining ½ teaspoon ginger. Blend in broth and soy sauce. Add to vegetable mixture. Add onions. Mix well. Microwave at High, uncovered, for 5 to 8 minutes, or until mixture thickens and bubbles, stirring 2 or 3 times. Cover to keep warm. Set aside.

Spray 12-inch nonstick skillet with nonstick vegetable cooking spray. Heat conventionally over medium-high heat. Add meat mixture. Cook for 5 to 7 minutes, or just until meat is no longer pink, turning over once. Drain. Add meat mixture and sour cream to casserole. Mix well. Serve immediately.

Serving suggestion: Serve over hot cooked Basmati rice.

*Substitute 1-lb. well-trimmed boneless beef sirloin steak for pork, if desired.

Per Serving: Calories: 303 • Protein: 32 g. • Carbohydrate: 21 g. • Fat: 12 g.
• Cholesterol: 83 mg. • Sodium: 719 mg.
Exchanges: ⅓ starch, 3 lean meat, 3 vegetable, ⅔ fat

Pork & Pasta Primavera ▶

8 oz. uncooked linguine
1 pkg. (9 oz.) frozen
    asparagus cuts
1 cup carrot strips
    (1½ × ¼-inch strips)
1 tablespoon water
1 cup thinly sliced red and
    yellow pepper strips
4 well-trimmed boneless
    pork sirloin chops (4 oz.
    each), ½ inch thick, cut
    into 1 × ¼-inch-thick strips
¼ cup all-purpose flour
1 teaspoon dried basil leaves
½ teaspoon salt
¼ teaspoon freshly ground
    pepper
1 clove garlic, minced
    Dash ground nutmeg
1½ cups whole milk
¼ cup sliced green onions
2 oz. freshly grated Parmesan
    cheese

4 servings

Prepare linguine as directed on package. Rinse and drain. Cover to keep warm. Set aside.

In 2-quart casserole, combine asparagus, carrots and water. Cover. Microwave at High for 8 to 11 minutes, or until carrots are tender, stirring twice. Add pepper strips. Cover to keep warm. Set aside.

Spray 12-inch nonstick skillet with nonstick vegetable cooking spray. Heat conventionally over medium-high heat. Add pork strips. Cook for 5 to 6 minutes, or just until meat is no longer pink, turning over once. Drain. Drain vegetables in casserole. Add meat to casserole. Cover to keep warm. Set aside.

In 4-cup measure, combine flour, basil, salt, pepper, garlic and nutmeg. Blend in milk. Microwave at High for 5 to 7 minutes, or until sauce thickens and bubbles, stirring after every minute. Pour sauce over vegetable and meat mixture. Add onions. Mix well. Cover. Microwave at High for 3 to 4 minutes, or until mixture is hot, stirring once. Spoon over linguine. Sprinkle evenly with Parmesan cheese.

Serving suggestion: Serve with spinach salad.

Per Serving: Calories: 536 • Protein: 43 g. • Carbohydrate: 61 g. • Fat: 15 g.
• Cholesterol: 96 mg. • Sodium: 613 mg.
Exchanges: 3 starch, 3½ lean meat, 2 vegetable, ½ skim milk, ½ fat

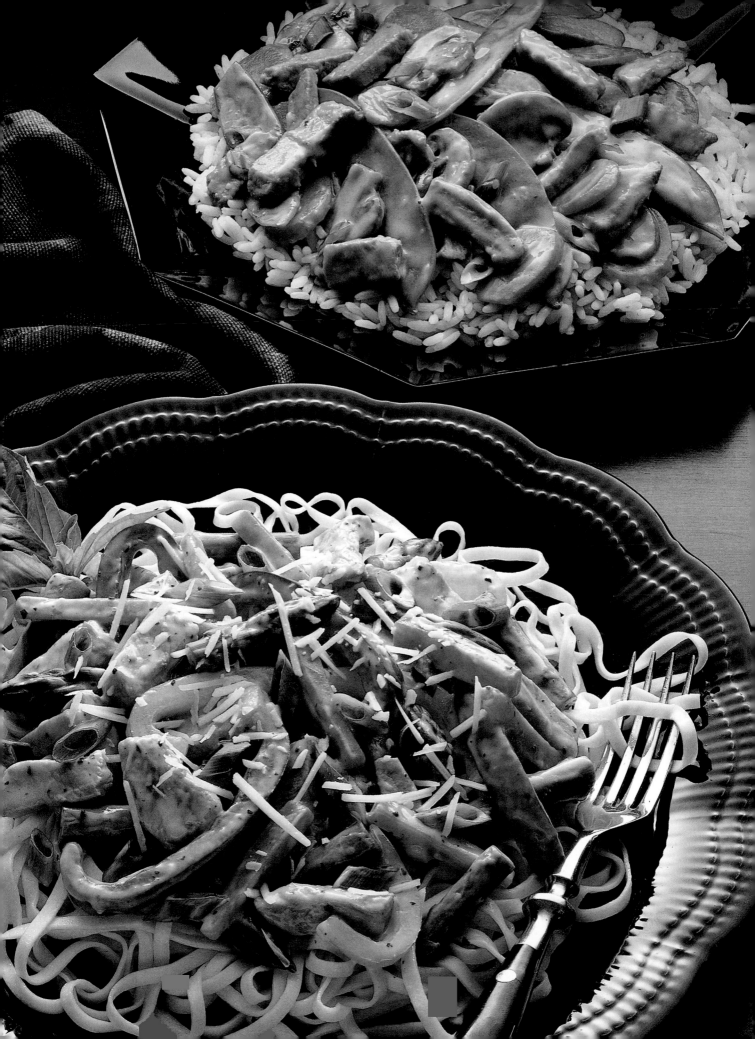

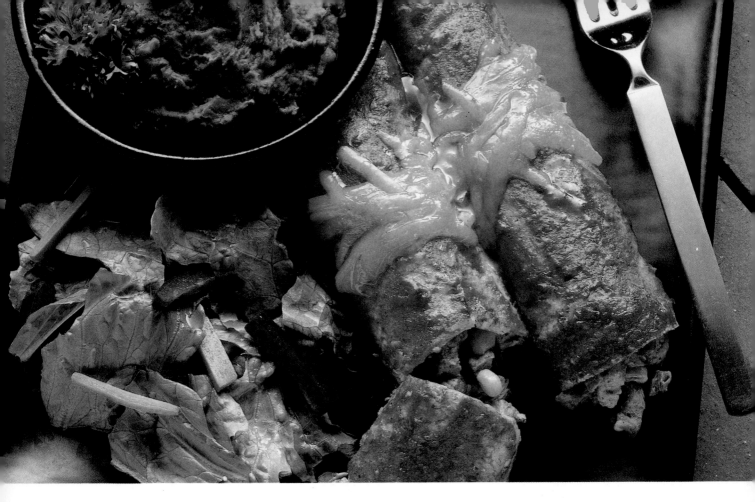

Spicy Pork Enchiladas

½ cup frozen corn
1 can (4 oz.) chopped green chilies
1 tablespoon water
1 teaspoon ground cumin, divided
1- lb. well-trimmed boneless pork top loin roast, cut into 1 × ¼-inch-thick strips
½ teaspoon chili powder
½ cup chopped onion
¾ cup grated reduced-fat Cheddar cheese (5 g. fat per oz.), divided
¼ cup light sour cream
¼ teaspoon salt
1 can (10 oz.) mild enchilada sauce, divided
8 corn tortillas (6-inch)

4 servings

Heat conventional oven to 350°F. In 2-cup measure, combine corn, green chilies, water and ½ teaspoon cumin. Microwave at High for 3 to 5 minutes, or until corn is hot, stirring once. Set aside.

Place pork strips in 2-quart casserole. Sprinkle with chili powder and remaining ½ teaspoon cumin. Toss to coat evenly. Add onion. Mix well. Cover. Microwave at High for 5 to 7 minutes, or just until meat is no longer pink, stirring once or twice. Drain. Add corn mixture, ½ cup cheese, the sour cream and salt. Mix well. Re-cover. Set aside. Spread ¼ cup enchilada sauce evenly in 11 × 7-inch baking dish. Set aside.

Place 4 tortillas between dampened paper towels. Microwave at High for 15 to 30 seconds, or until tortillas are warm. Repeat for remaining tortillas. Place ⅓ cup of meat mixture down center of each tortilla. Roll up and place seam-side-down in prepared baking dish. Pour remaining sauce evenly over enchiladas. Top with remaining ¼ cup cheese. Cover with foil. Bake conventionally for 15 minutes. Remove foil. Bake for 5 to 10 minutes longer, or until cheese is melted and sauce is hot and bubbly.

Serving suggestion: Serve with tossed green salad and spicy refried beans.

Per Serving: Calories: 462 • Protein: 40 g. • Carbohydrate: 42 g. • Fat: 15 g.
• Cholesterol: 88 mg. • Sodium: 1305 mg.
Exchanges: 2 starch, 4 lean meat, 1 vegetable, ¼ skim milk, ½ fat

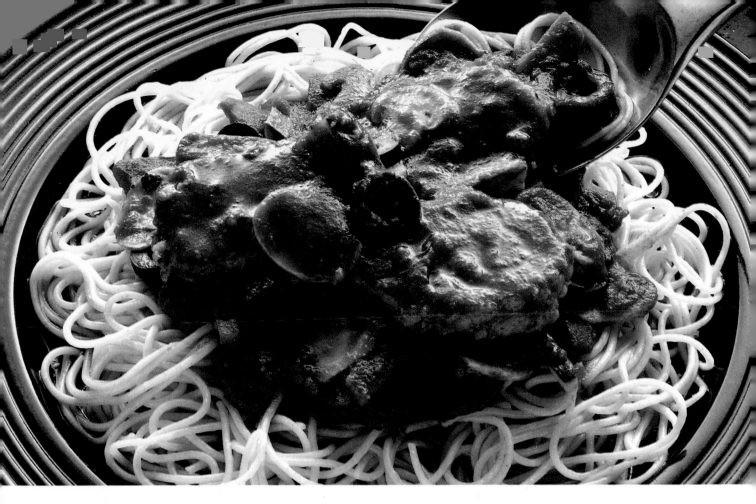

Pork Cacciatore

6 oz. fresh mushrooms, sliced
   (1½ cups)
½ cup chopped onion
1 medium carrot, cut into
   1 × ¼-inch strips (½ cup)
2 cloves garlic, minced
1 tablespoon plus 1 teaspoon
   olive oil, divided
1 can (14½ oz.) diced
   tomatoes, undrained
1 can (8 oz.) tomato sauce
1 small zucchini, cut into
   1 × ⅛-inch strips (½ cup)
¼ cup sliced black olives
1 teaspoon dried oregano
   leaves
1 bay leaf
½ teaspoon salt, divided
½ teaspoon freshly ground
   pepper, divided
¼ cup all-purpose flour
1 well-trimmed pork
   tenderloin (approx. 1 lb.),
   cut crosswise into 8 pieces
1 pkg. (7 oz.) uncooked
   vermicelli

4 servings

In 2-quart casserole, combine mushrooms, onion, carrot, garlic and 2 teaspoons oil. Cover. Microwave at High for 5 to 7 minutes, or until onion is tender, stirring once. Add tomatoes, tomato sauce, zucchini, olives, oregano, bay leaf, ¼ teaspoon salt and ¼ teaspoon pepper. Mix well. Cover. Set aside.

In shallow dish, combine flour and remaining ¼ teaspoon each salt and pepper. Pound pork pieces lightly to ¼-inch thickness. Dredge in flour mixture, turning to coat both sides. In 12-inch nonstick skillet, heat 1 teaspoon oil conventionally over medium-high heat. Add 4 pork pieces. Cook for 5 to 6 minutes, or just until meat is no longer pink, turning over once. Place on plate. Cover to keep warm. Set aside. Repeat with remaining 1 teaspoon oil and pork pieces.

Spoon half of vegetable mixture into 10-inch square casserole. Arrange pork pieces in single layer over vegetables. Top with remaining vegetable mixture. Cover. Microwave at High for 5 minutes. Microwave at 50% (Medium) for 10 to 15 minutes longer, or until sauce is hot and flavors are blended, stirring once. Let stand for 5 minutes. Prepare vermicelli as directed on package. Serve cacciatore over vermicelli.

Serving suggestion: Serve with tossed green salad.

Per Serving: Calories: 468 • Protein: 34 g. • Carbohydrate: 59 g. • Fat: 11 g.
• Cholesterol: 74 mg. • Sodium: 926 mg.
Exchanges: 2½ starch, 3 lean meat, 3 vegetable, ½ fat

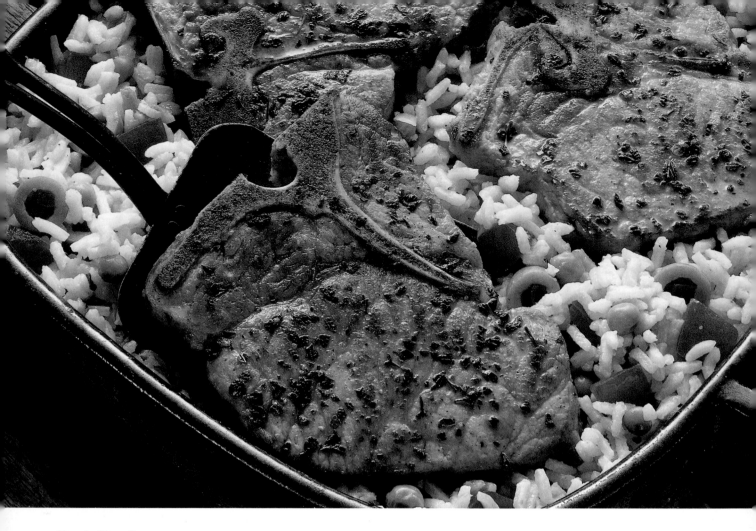

Pork Paella

Seasoning Mixture:

- 1 teaspoon dried oregano leaves
- ½ teaspoon garlic powder
- ½ teaspoon salt
- ¼ teaspoon freshly ground pepper

- 1¼ cups uncooked long-grain white rice
- ½ cup chopped onion
- 3 tablespoons canned chopped green chilies
- ¼ teaspoon saffron
- 1 can (14½ oz.) ready-to-serve chicken broth
- ½ cup water
- 1 medium tomato, seeded and chopped
- ½ cup frozen peas
- ¼ cup halved pimiento-stuffed green olives
- 4 well-trimmed bone-in pork center loin or rib chops (8 oz. each), 1 inch thick

4 servings

In small bowl, combine seasoning mixture ingredients. Set aside. In 10-inch square casserole, combine rice, onion, chilies, saffron, broth, water and 1 teaspoon seasoning mixture. Cover. Microwave at High for 8 minutes. Microwave at 50% (Medium) for 15 to 20 minutes longer, or until rice is tender and liquid is absorbed. Let stand, covered, for 5 minutes. Add tomato, peas and olives. Cover. Set aside.

Sprinkle both sides of pork chops evenly with remaining seasoning mixture. Spray 10-inch nonstick skillet with nonstick vegetable cooking spray. Heat skillet conventionally over medium-high heat. Add chops. Cook for 5 to 6 minutes, or just until meat is browned on both sides. Arrange chops over rice mixture with meaty portions toward outside. Cover. Microwave at 70% (Medium High) for 15 to 18 minutes, or just until meat is no longer pink, turning chops over once.

Serving suggestion: Serve with mixed tropical fruit salad or tossed green salad.

Per Serving: Calories: 451 • Protein: 35 g. • Carbohydrate: 54 g. • Fat: 11 g. • Cholesterol: 78 mg. • Sodium: 1064 mg.
Exchanges: 3 starch, 3 lean meat, 2 vegetable, ½ fat

Pork Chops Marengo

4 well-trimmed bone-in pork
    rib or center loin chops
    (8 oz. each), 1 inch thick
1 teaspoon paprika
1 tablespoon olive oil
2 cloves garlic, minced
1 can (16 oz.) whole tomatoes,
    undrained and cut up
4 oz. fresh mushrooms, sliced
    (1 cup)
⅓ cup sliced green onions
¼ cup sliced black olives
2 tablespoons tomato paste
1 tablespoon brandy (optional)
½ teaspoon dried thyme leaves
1 bay leaf
½ teaspoon sugar

4 servings

Sprinkle both sides of pork chops
evenly with paprika. Set aside.
In 12-inch nonstick skillet, heat
oil conventionally over medium-
high heat. Add garlic. Sauté for
1 minute, or until tender. Add
chops. Cook for 5 to 6 minutes,
or just until meat is browned on
both sides. Arrange chops in 10-
inch square casserole. Set aside.

In medium mixing bowl, combine
remaining ingredients. Spoon
over chops. Cover. Microwave
at 70% (Medium High) for 10 to
15 minutes, or just until meat is
no longer pink, turning chops
over and rotating casserole twice.

Serving suggestion: Serve with
hot cooked rice.

Per Serving: Calories: 267 • Protein: 30 g.
• Carbohydrate: 10 g. • Fat: 14 g.
• Cholesterol: 78 mg. • Sodium: 398 mg.
Exchanges: 3 lean meat, 2 vegetable, 1 fat

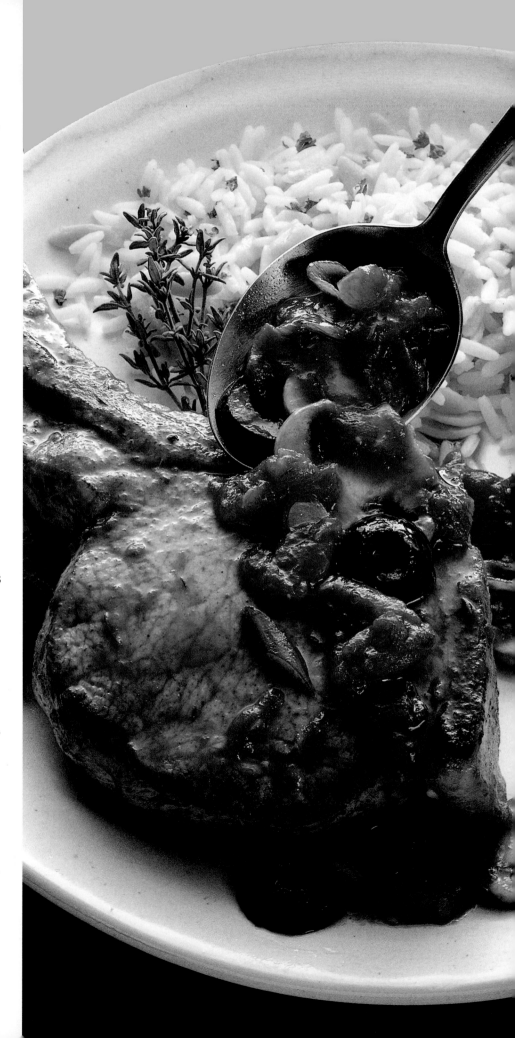

Pork & Pear Pie

- 1 cup chopped onions
- 1 tablespoon margarine or butter
- 2 cups cubed red potatoes (1/2-inch cubes)
- 1 cup carrot strips (1 × 1/4-inch strips)
- 2 tablespoons water
- 1 1/2-lb. well-trimmed boneless pork top loin roast, cut into 1/2-inch cubes

- 2 pears, cored and cut into 1/2-inch cubes
- 2 tablespoons all-purpose flour, divided
- 3/4 cup plain nonfat yogurt
- 1 teaspoon packed brown sugar
- 1 teaspoon ground sage
- 1 teaspoon salt
- 1/8 teaspoon pepper
- 1 oz. blue cheese, crumbled

- 1 cup buttermilk baking mix
- 1/4 cup skim milk

6 servings

Serving suggestion: Serve with fresh fruit salad.

Per Serving: Calories: 406 • Protein: 33 g. • Carbohydrate: 39 g. • Fat: 13 g. • Cholesterol: 73 mg. • Sodium: 782 mg. Exchanges: 2 starch, 3 lean meat, 1 vegetable, 1/4 skim milk, 1 fat

How to Make Pork & Pear Pie

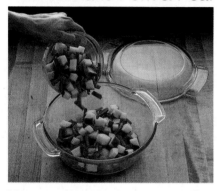

Heat conventional oven to 450°F. Place onions and margarine in 2-quart casserole. Cover. Microwave at High for 4 to 6 minutes, or until onions are tender-crisp, stirring once. Add potatoes, carrots and water. Mix well. Re-cover.

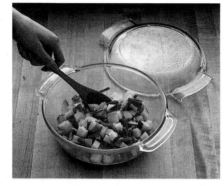

Microwave at High for 9 to 11 minutes, or until potatoes are tender, stirring once or twice. Cover to keep warm. Set aside. Spray 12-inch nonstick skillet with nonstick vegetable cooking spray. Heat conventionally over medium-high heat.

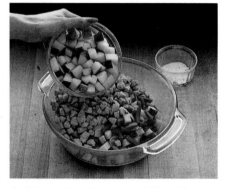

Add pork cubes to skillet. Cook for 7 to 9 minutes, or just until meat is no longer pink, stirring once or twice. Drain. Add pork and pears to vegetable mixture. Sprinkle 1 tablespoon flour over mixture. Mix well. Cover to keep warm. Set aside.

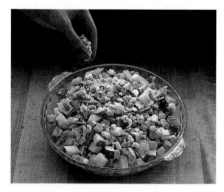

Combine yogurt, sugar, sage, salt and pepper in 2-cup measure. Pour over pork and pear mixture. Mix well. Spoon mixture into 10-inch deep-dish pie plate. Sprinkle blue cheese evenly over top. Cover with foil to keep warm. Set aside.

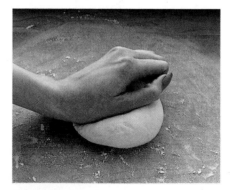

Combine baking mix and milk in medium mixing bowl. Stir just until mixture is moistened and clings together. Sprinkle remaining 1 tablespoon flour over work surface. Turn out dough onto work surface and knead 3 or 4 times, or until dough is smooth.

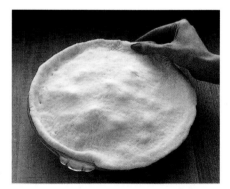

Roll dough into 12-inch circle. Remove foil from pie. Place dough over pie. Roll edges of dough under and against sides of pie plate to seal. Cut several slits in crust. Bake conventionally for 10 to 12 minutes, or until crust is lightly browned.

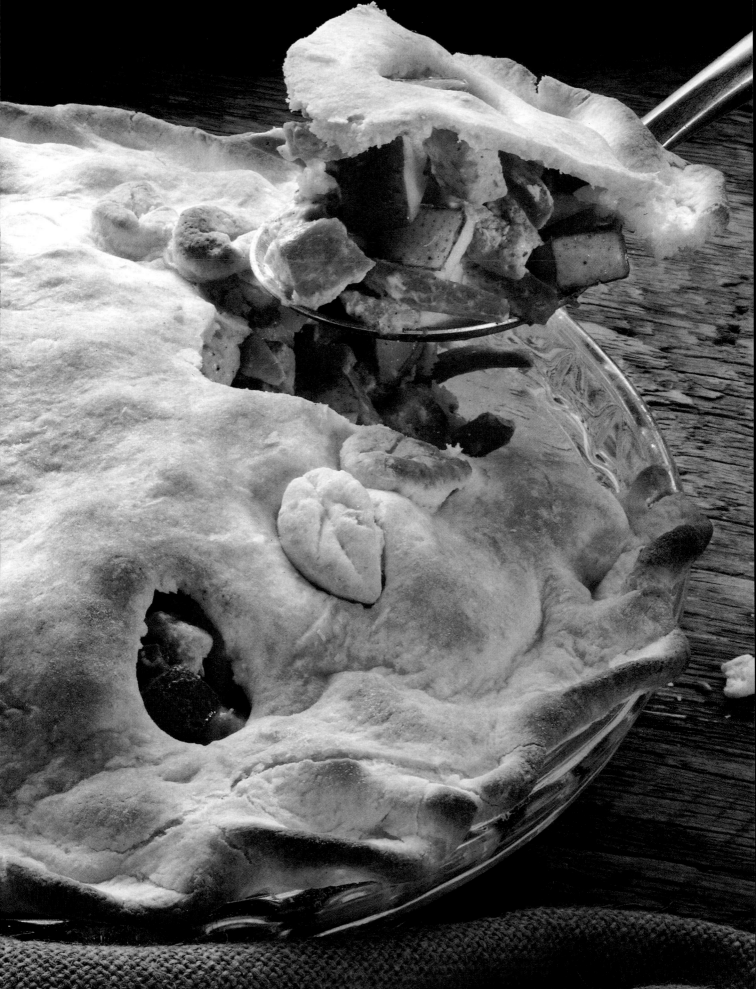

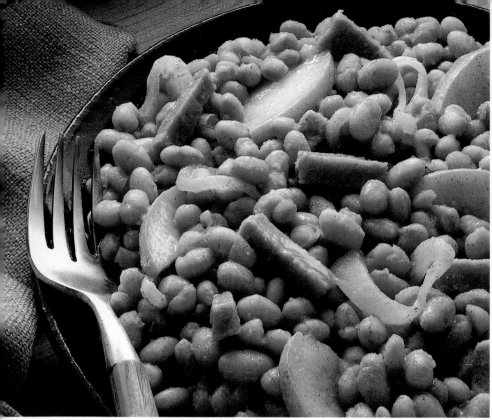

Spicy Barbecued Pork Loin Sandwiches

1 medium onion, thinly sliced
1 medium green pepper, cut
  into thin strips
2 teaspoons vegetable oil
1 can (8 oz.) tomato sauce
¼ cup red wine vinegar
¼ cup packed brown sugar
1 tablespoon tomato paste
2½ teaspoons chili powder
1 teaspoon reduced-sodium
  Worcestershire sauce
1 teaspoon salt

1 teaspoon garlic powder
½ teaspoon ground ginger
½ teaspoon freshly ground
  pepper
¼ teaspoon cayenne
¼ teaspoon ground cloves
2-lb. well-trimmed
  boneless pork single loin
  roast
8 sesame seed buns, split
  and toasted

8 servings

Heat conventional oven to 350°F. In 1-quart casserole, combine onion, green pepper and oil. Cover. Microwave at High for 5 to 7 minutes, or until onion is tender-crisp, stirring once. Add remaining ingredients, except pork and buns. Mix well. Set sauce aside.

Place pork in 11 × 7-inch baking dish. Cover with wax paper or microwave cooking paper. Microwave at 70% (Medium High) for 7 to 9 minutes, or just until edges are no longer pink, turning over once. Pour sauce over meat. Bake conventionally, uncovered, for 50 minutes to 1 hour, or until internal temperature registers 155°F and juices run clear. Let stand, tented with foil, for 10 minutes. (Internal temperature will rise 5°F during standing.) Carve meat across grain into thin slices. Return meat to baking dish. Spoon sauce over meat. Serve hot on buns.

Serving suggestion: Serve with black bean and corn salad.

Per Serving: Calories: 361 • Protein: 30 g. • Carbohydrate: 36 g. • Fat: 11 g.
• Cholesterol: 65 mg. • Sodium: 730 mg.
Exchanges: 1½ starch, 3 lean meat, 1 vegetable, ½ fruit, ½ fat

◄ Maple-Apple Baked Ham & Beans

½ cup sliced onion
1 tablespoon margarine or
  butter
2 cans (15½ oz. each) navy
  beans, rinsed and drained
1 medium Rome or Granny
  Smith apple (or half of
  each), cored and cut into
  ⅛-inch slices
⅓ cup pure maple syrup
1 tablespoon plus 1 teaspoon
  apple cider vinegar
1 teaspoon dark molasses
½ teaspoon dry mustard
½ teaspoon ground cinnamon
¾ lb. fully cooked boneless
  ham, cut into 1 × ¼-inch
  strips

4 servings

In 2-quart casserole, microwave onion and margarine at High for 3 to 4 minutes, or until onion is tender-crisp, stirring once. Add remaining ingredients, except ham strips. Microwave at High, uncovered, for 8 to 10 minutes, or until beans are hot and apple is tender-crisp, stirring 2 or 3 times. Add ham. Microwave at High for 3 to 5 minutes, or until mixture is hot, stirring once.

Serving suggestion: Serve with warm corn bread wedges or buttermilk biscuits.

Per Serving: Calories: 421 • Protein: 30 g.
• Carbohydrate: 56 g. • Fat: 9 g.
• Cholesterol: 45 mg. • Sodium: 1335 mg.
Exchanges: 2 starch, 3 lean meat, 1¾ fruit

Savory Ham & Cabbage Strudel

4 cups shredded green cabbage
1/4 cup water
1/2 cup shredded carrot
1/2 cup sliced green onions
1/3 cup light sour cream
1 teaspoon caraway seed
3/4 lb. fully cooked boneless ham, cut into 1/2-inch cubes
1/4 cup margarine or butter
12 sheets frozen phyllo dough (18 × 14-inch sheets), defrosted

4 servings

Heat conventional oven to 375°F. In 2-quart casserole, combine cabbage and water. Cover. Microwave at High for 6 to 10 minutes, or until cabbage is tender, stirring once. Drain, pressing to remove excess moisture. Return to casserole. Stir in carrot, onions, sour cream, caraway seed and ham cubes. Set filling aside.

In small bowl, microwave margarine at High for 1 1/4 to 1 1/2 minutes, or until melted. Unroll phyllo sheets. Cover with plastic wrap. Working quickly, place 1 sheet of phyllo on work surface. Brush lightly with margarine. Top with another sheet of phyllo. Brush lightly with margarine. Repeat with remaining sheets of phyllo, forming layers.

Spoon filling lengthwise down center of phyllo sheets to within 2 inches of short ends and 4 inches of long sides. Fold long sides of phyllo over filling. Fold ends under to seal. Place strudel seam-side-down on large baking sheet. Bake for 25 to 30 minutes, or until golden brown. Serve immediately.

Serving suggestion: Serve with assorted fresh fruits.

Per Serving: Calories: 475 • Protein: 27 g.
• Carbohydrate: 49 g. • Fat: 20 g.
• Cholesterol: 52 mg. • Sodium: 1428 mg.
Exchanges: 2 1/2 starch, 3 lean meat, 2 vegetable, 1 1/2 fat

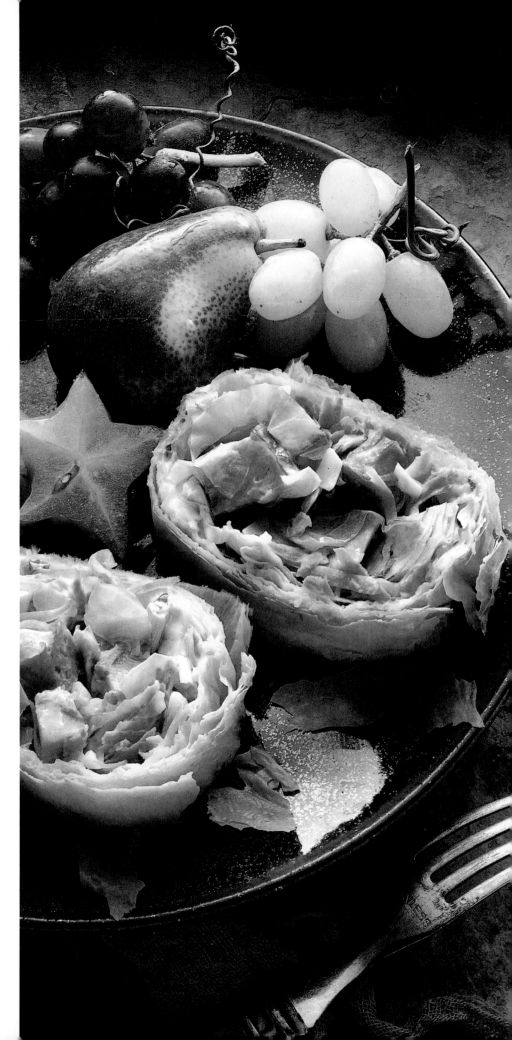

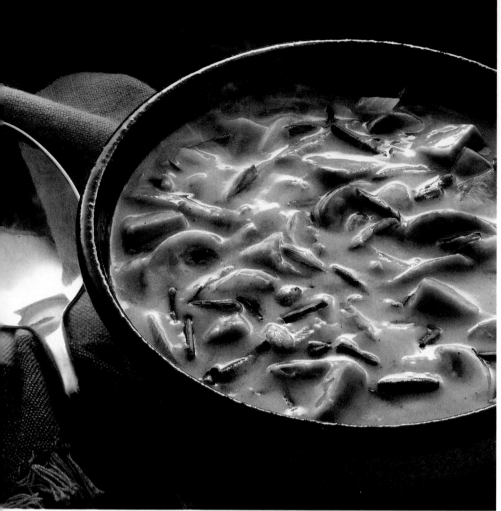

Curried Ham & Wild Rice Stew

- 1 cup chopped onions
- 3 tablespoons margarine or butter
- 12 oz. fresh mushrooms, sliced (3 cups)
- ½ cup sliced celery
- ½ cup all-purpose flour
- 2 cans (14½ oz. each) low-sodium ready-to-serve chicken broth
- 1 teaspoon curry powder
- ¼ teaspoon dry mustard
- ¼ teaspoon paprika
- ¼ teaspoon white pepper
- ¾ lb. fully cooked boneless ham, cut into ½-inch cubes
- 2 cups cooked wild rice
- 1 cup whole milk
- ½ cup grated carrot
- ¼ cup dry sherry

4 servings

Place onions and margarine in 3-quart casserole. Cover. Microwave at High for 4 to 6 minutes, or until onions are tender-crisp, stirring once. Add mushrooms and celery. Mix well. Re-cover. Microwave at High for 4 to 6 minutes, or until celery is tender-crisp, stirring once.

Stir in flour. Blend in broth. Add curry, mustard, paprika and pepper. Mix well. Re-cover. Microwave at High for 12 to 17 minutes, or until mixture thickens slightly and bubbles, stirring 2 or 3 times. Add remaining ingredients. Mix well. Re-cover. Microwave at High for 7 to 9 minutes, or until soup is hot, stirring once.

Serving suggestion: Serve with soft bread sticks and tossed green salad.

Per Serving: Calories: 458 • Protein: 29 g.
• Carbohydrate: 46 g. • Fat: 18 g.
• Cholesterol: 54 mg. • Sodium: 1229 mg.
Exchanges: 2 starch, 3 lean meat,
1 vegetable, ¼ skim milk, 1¾ fat

Sherried Split Pea & Ham Soup

- ½ cup chopped onion
- ½ cup chopped celery
- 1 tablespoon vegetable oil
- 4 cups hot water
- 1 cup dried split peas
- 2 bay leaves
- 1 cup cubed red potatoes (¾-inch cubes)
- ¾ cup thinly sliced carrot
- ¾ teaspoon dried basil leaves
- ½ teaspoon dried thyme leaves
- ¾ lb. fully cooked boneless ham, cut into 1 × ¼-inch-thick strips
- ¼ cup dry sherry

4 servings

In 2-quart casserole, combine onion, celery and oil. Microwave at High for 5 to 7 minutes, or until onion is tender, stirring once. Add water, split peas and bay leaves. Mix well. Cover. Microwave at High for 10 minutes. Microwave at 50% (Medium) for 40 minutes longer, stirring once.

Add potatoes, carrot, basil and thyme. Mix well. Cover. Microwave at 50% (Medium) for 25 to 35 minutes, or until peas are tender, stirring once. Stir in ham. Cover. Microwave at 50% (Medium) for 2 to 3 minutes, or until mixture is hot, stirring once. Before serving, remove and discard bay leaves. Blend in sherry.

Serving suggestion: Serve with warm whole-grain rolls.

Per Serving: Calories: 396 • Protein: 31 g. • Carbohydrate: 44 g. • Fat: 9 g.
• Cholesterol: 45 mg. • Sodium: 1057 mg.
Exchanges: 2½ starch, 3 lean meat, 1¼ vegetable

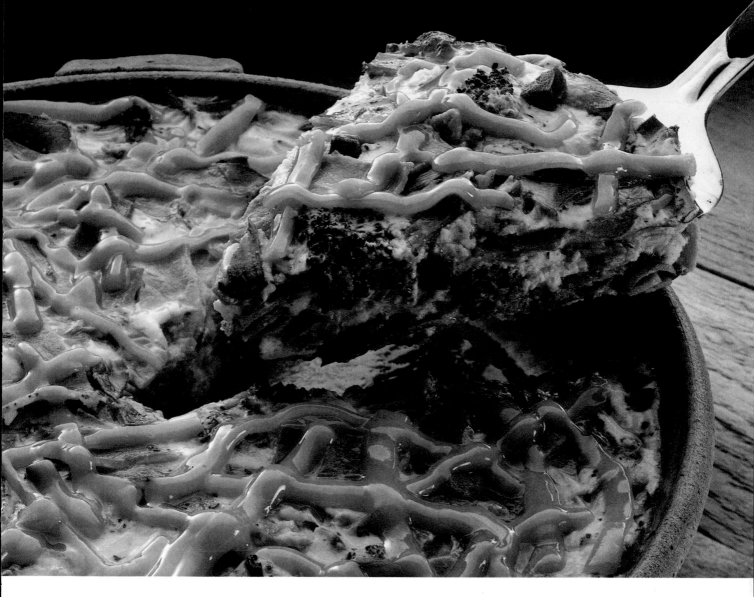

Crustless Canadian-style Bacon & Broccoli Quiche

1 ½ cups frozen broccoli cuts
   and red pepper
1 tablespoon water
1 carton (8 oz.) Egg
   Beaters®, defrosted
1 cup 2% milk
⅓ cup sliced green onions
2 tablespoons all-purpose
   flour
½ teaspoon dried basil leaves
½ teaspoon dried marjoram
   leaves
¼ teaspoon salt
¼ teaspoon pepper
¾ lb. Canadian-style bacon
   slices, cut into 1 × ½-inch-
   thick strips
1 cup shredded reduced-fat
   Cheddar cheese (5 g. fat
   per oz.), divided

6 servings

Heat conventional oven to 350°F. Spray 9-inch pie plate with nonstick vegetable cooking spray. Set aside. Chop broccoli mixture into small pieces. In 2-quart casserole, combine broccoli mixture and water. Cover. Microwave at High for 4 to 6 minutes, or until hot, stirring once. Drain, pressing to remove excess moisture. Return to casserole.

Add remaining ingredients, except bacon and cheese. Mix well. Microwave at 50% (Medium), uncovered, for 8 to 13 minutes, or until mixture is hot and edges just begin to set, stirring every 2 minutes. Add bacon and ¾ cup cheese. Mix well. Pour into prepared dish. Sprinkle remaining ¼ cup cheese evenly over top. Bake conventionally for 25 to 30 minutes, or until quiche is set and knife inserted in center comes out clean. Let stand for 10 minutes.

Serving suggestion: Serve with melon wedges and whole fresh strawberries.

Per Serving: Calories: 214 • Protein: 23 g. • Carbohydrate: 9 g. • Fat: 8 g.
• Cholesterol: 45 mg. • Sodium: 1108 mg.
Exchanges: 3 lean meat, 1 vegetable

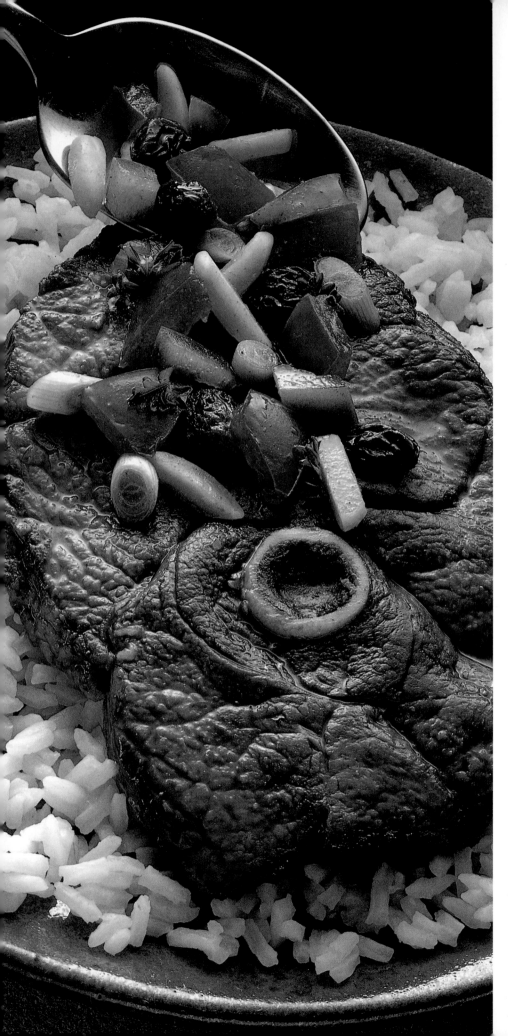

Lamb & Veal

Lamb Steaks with Curry Salsa

½ cup raisins
½ cup water
2 cups seeded chopped tomatoes
½ cup chopped green pepper
½ cup sliced green onions
¼ cup slivered almonds
¼ cup snipped fresh parsley
2 teaspoons curry powder
2 well-trimmed bone-in lamb leg steaks (¾ lb. each), ¾ inch thick

6 servings

Place raisins and water in 2-cup measure. Cover with plastic wrap. Microwave at High for 2 to 3 minutes, or until water begins to boil and raisins are plumped. Let stand for 5 minutes. Drain.

In medium mixing bowl, combine raisins, tomatoes, green pepper, onions, almonds, parsley and curry powder. Cover and refrigerate salsa at least 1 hour.

Arrange steaks on rack in broiler pan. Place under conventional broiler, with surface of meat 3 to 4 inches from heat. Broil for 10 to 12 minutes, or until desired doneness, turning once. Cut steaks into serving-size pieces. Top with salsa.

Serving suggestion: Serve with hot cooked rice.

Per Serving: Calories: 262 • Protein: 26 g.
• Carbohydrate: 15 g. • Fat: 11 g.
• Cholesterol: 78 mg. • Sodium: 69 mg.
Exchanges: 3 lean meat, 1½ vegetable, ½ fruit, ½ fat

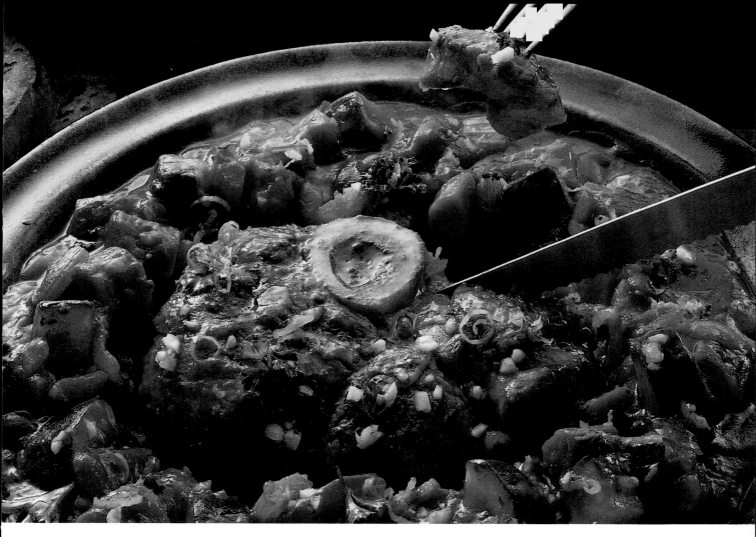

Osso Buco

    3   tablespoons all-purpose flour, divided
    1   cup chopped celery
    1   cup chopped carrots
    ½   cup chopped onion
    3   tablespoons tomato paste
    1   tablespoon fresh thyme leaves or
          1 teaspoon dried thyme leaves
    ½   teaspoon salt
    1   cup ready-to-serve beef broth
    ½   cup dry white wine
    1   tablespoon olive oil
    2¼ lbs. veal shank crosscuts, cut 1 inch thick
    1   medium tomato, seeded and chopped
    1   cup chopped zucchini

Topping:
    2   tablespoons snipped fresh parsley
    1   tablespoon grated lemon peel
    1   or 2 cloves garlic, minced

                                   4 servings

Place 1 tablespoon flour in large oven cooking bag. Hold bag closed at top and shake to coat. Add celery, carrots, onion, remaining 2 tablespoons flour, the tomato paste, thyme and salt. Mix well. Blend in broth and wine. Place bag in 10-inch square casserole. Set aside.

In 12-inch nonstick skillet, heat oil conventionally over medium-high heat. Add veal shanks. Cook for 5 to 7 minutes, or just until meat is browned on both sides. Remove from heat. Add shanks to vegetable mixture in bag. Secure bag with nylon tie. Make six ½-inch slits in neck of bag below tie. Microwave at 50% (Medium) for 45 minutes. Turn shanks over. Add tomato and zucchini. Secure bag. Microwave at 50% (Medium) for 15 to 30 minutes, or until meat is tender. Let bag stand, closed, for 10 minutes.

In small bowl, combine topping ingredients. Sprinkle evenly over each serving of Osso Buco.

Serving suggestion: Serve with crusty French bread or risotto.

Per Serving: Calories: 289 • Protein: 39 g. • Carbohydrate: 17 g.
• Fat: 7 g. • Cholesterol: 130 mg. • Sodium: 728 mg.
Exchanges: ¼ starch, 4 lean meat, 2½ vegetable

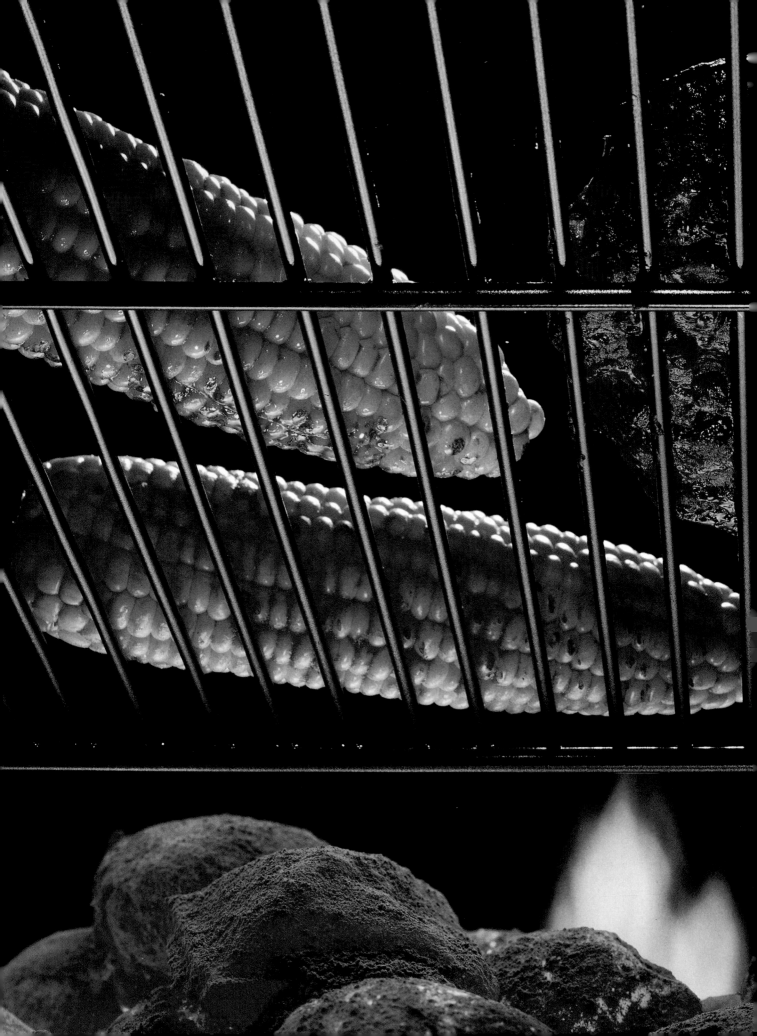

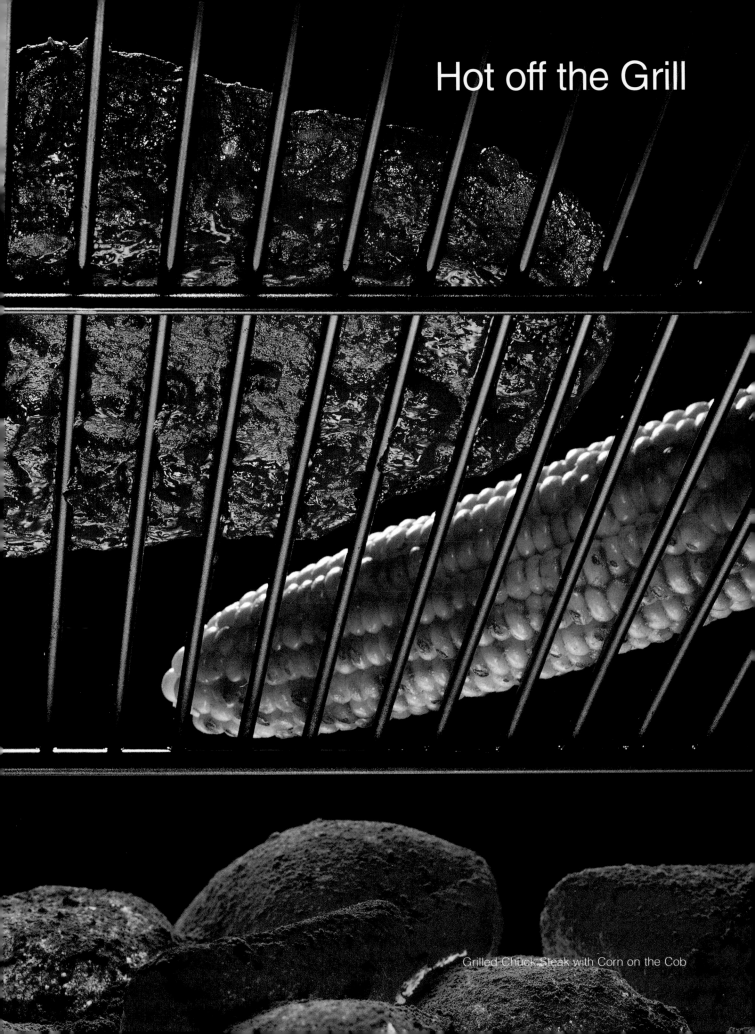

Hot off the Grill

Grilled Chuck Steak with Corn on the Cob

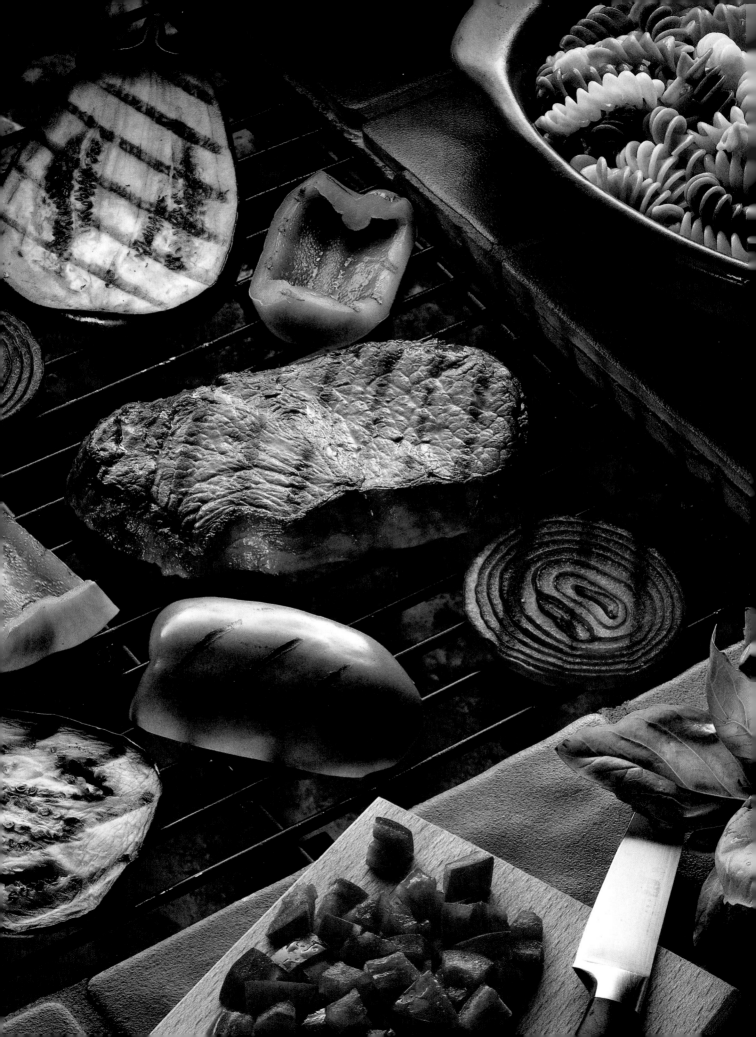

Barbecue Basics

Grilling lean meat without added fat is an ideal cooking method for a low-fat life-style. To flavor, tenderize and moisten meat during cooking, use one of the low-fat marinades in this section.

With cuts identified as intermediate/tender in the chart on pages 8 to 13, take care that the meat doesn't dry out and toughen. For the best results, grill these meats to rare or medium-rare.

Grilling Utensils

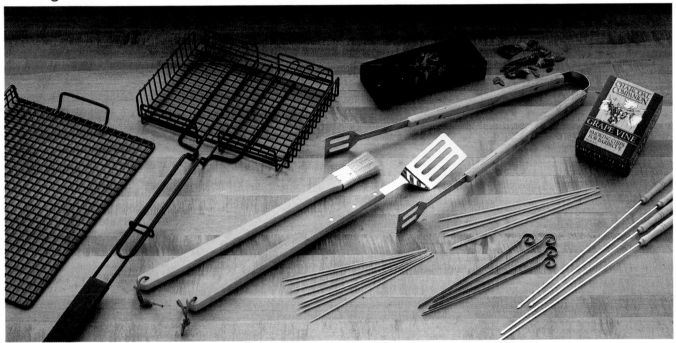

Left to right: Screens and baskets keep small items from falling through the cooking grid onto coals. Long-handled tongs, spatula and basting brush protect hands from heat. For kabobs, choose metal skewers, or soak wooden skewers in water for 20 to 30 minutes before assembling kabobs. To add smoky flavor and aroma to grilled meats, soak fragrant fruit-wood chips in water. Place in smoker box prior to grilling, or use smoker log (below).

How to Make a Smoker Log

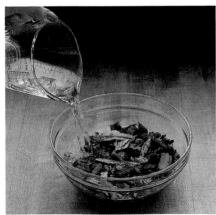

Soak 2 cups smoking chips in 4 cups water for 1 hour. Drain on paper towels.

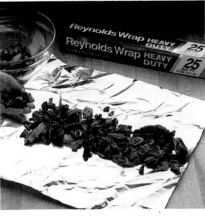

Place chips in center of 16-inch-long sheet of heavy-duty foil. Bring edges of foil together.

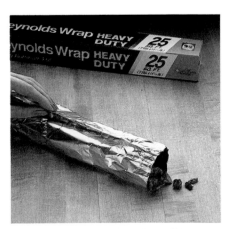

Fold down to make log. Place log directly on hot coals.

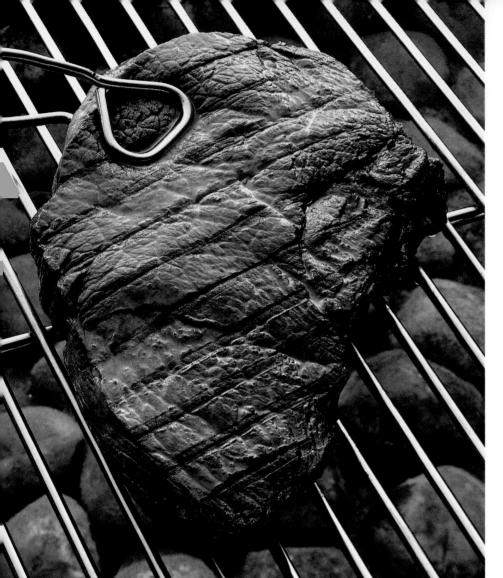

Grilling Methods

Whether you use a charcoal or gas grill, there are two methods of barbecuing meat: direct heat or indirect heat. Small cuts such as steaks, chops, kabobs or burgers can be grilled quickly over *direct heat*. Large cuts like roasts need a longer cooking time and should be prepared over *indirect heat* on a covered grill.

Micro-grilling, partial cooking in the microwave oven just before placing the meat on the grill, ensures that the meat will be fully cooked but still juicy inside by the time the grill gives it a rich color and barbecue flavor. Micro-grilled meats cook faster and don't dry out. Microwave the meat ten minutes before the grill reaches cooking temperature. Take the meat directly from the microwave oven to the grill.

Direct-heat Grilling. Use enough charcoal or lava rocks to spread under the meat and 1 inch beyond. Stack charcoal in a pyramid to light fire; when a light covering of ash forms (in about 30 minutes), spread coals out again. Preheat a gas grill for about 10 minutes on high setting.

Indirect Charcoal Grilling.
Place foil drip pan in center or to one side of grate. Heap charcoal beside it. When coals are hot, arrange food on cooking grid directly over drip pan. To maintain temperature, add a few more pieces of charcoal every 30 to 45 minutes.

Indirect Gas Grilling. Remove cooking grid. Preheat grill on high setting for 10 minutes, using all burners. Place foil drip pan on lava rocks in center or on one side of grate. With 2 or 3-burner grill, turn off burner under drip pan. Replace grid and arrange food over drip pan.

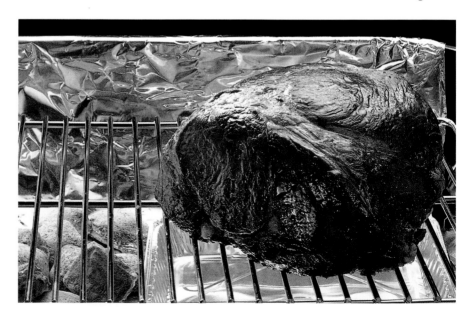

Judging Grill Temperature

Regulate the gas grill as you would a stove burner, setting it at high, medium or low. Check the temperature of a charcoal fire by extending the palm of your hand about 4 inches above the coals. Count the seconds before heat forces your hand away: 2 seconds, HOT; 3 seconds, MEDIUM-HOT; 4 seconds, MEDIUM; 5 seconds, LOW.

The appearance of the coals also indicates temperature. Once the coals develop a light coating of gray ash, the fire is HOT. A heavier layer of ash, with coals glowing through it, means the fire is MEDIUM. A thick layer of ash insulates the coals and reduces temperature to LOW.

Controlling Heat

With a gas grill, turn the temperature setting up or down to control heat. Use a higher setting on cold or windy days.

You can reduce the cooking temperature of a charcoal grill by spreading out the coals. To increase heat, tap the ash off the coals and move them closer together.

On a covered grill, open vents allow more air flow, which raises temperature. Partially close the vents to reduce heat.

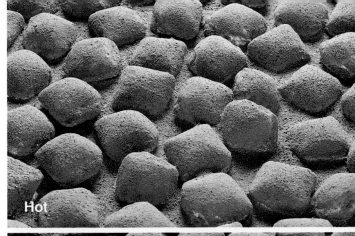

Hot

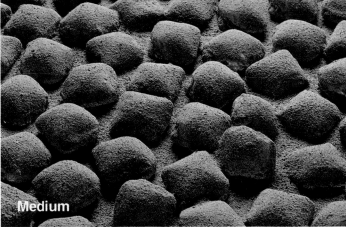

Medium

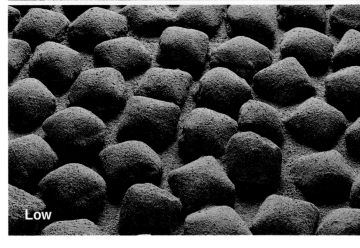

Low

Food Safety Tips for Grilled Meats

In addition to daily food safety practices, such as washing hands, utensils and cutting boards with hot soapy water before and after contact with uncooked meats, here are a few with special application to grilling:

- Refrigerate meat or keep it in insulated cooler until ready to grill.
- Always marinate meat in the refrigerator, not at room temperature.
- If marinade is to be used as a sauce, reserve some marinade and add meat to the remainder. Drain and do not reuse marinade from meat.

- Use separate platters for carrying raw and cooked meats, or line your platter with wax paper to carry raw meat. When meat is on the grill, discard paper and use clean platter for cooked meat.
- Do not interrupt cooking. Partial cooking may encourage bacterial growth during the delay. When micro-grilling, take meat to grill immediately after microwaving.
- Freeze or refrigerate leftover grilled meat promptly.

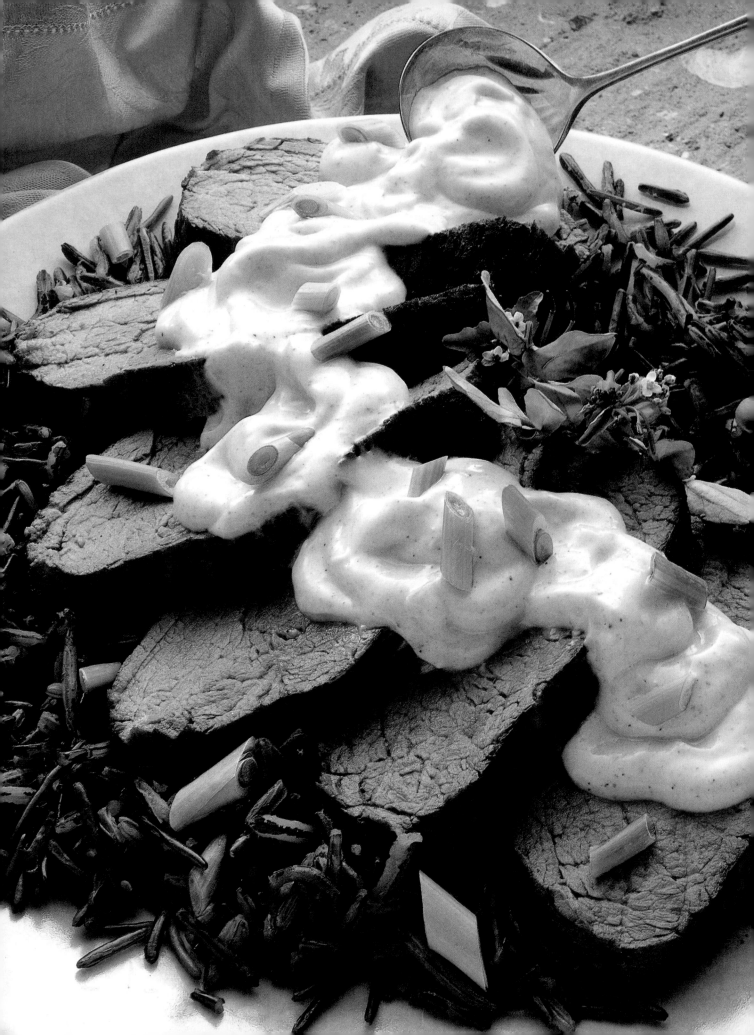

Beef

◄ Elegant Beef Tenderloin with Curry Sauce

1 - lb. well-trimmed beef
    tenderloin
1/4 cup finely chopped onion
1 teaspoon vegetable oil
1/2 teaspoon curry powder
2 tablespoons water
3/4 cup light sour cream
1/2 teaspoon lemon juice
2 tablespoons sliced green
    onion

4 servings

Spray cooking grid with nonstick vegetable cooking spray. Prepare grill for medium direct heat. Place tenderloin on cooking grid. Grill, covered, for 18 to 24 minutes for rare (135°F) to medium (155°F), or to desired doneness, turning occasionally. Remove meat from grill. Cover to keep warm. (Internal temperature will rise 5°F during standing.) Set aside.

In small mixing bowl, combine chopped onion and oil. Microwave at High for 1 1/2 to 3 minutes, or until onion is tender, stirring once. Add curry powder and water. Microwave at High for 2 to 3 minutes, or just until water has evaporated. Stir in sour cream and juice. Microwave at High for 1 to 1 1/2 minutes, or until sauce is warm. Carve meat across grain into thin slices. Spoon sauce over meat. Sprinkle with green onion.

Serving suggestion: Serve on bed of hot cooked wild rice.

Per Serving: Calories: 257 • Protein: 27 g.
• Carbohydrate: 7 g. • Fat: 13 g.
• Cholesterol: 72 mg. • Sodium: 114 mg.
Exchanges: 3 lean meat, 1 1/2 vegetable,
3/4 fat

Butterflied Eye Round Roast with Horseradish Sauce

Horseradish Sauce:
1/2 cup reduced-calorie
    mayonnaise
1/4 cup snipped fresh parsley
1/4 cup snipped fresh chives
1 tablespoon prepared
    horseradish

Marinade:
1/3 cup chopped onion

2 tablespoons vegetable oil
1 clove garlic, minced
1/4 cup red wine vinegar
1 tablespoon prepared
    horseradish
1/4 teaspoon crushed red
    pepper flakes

2 - lb. beef eye round roast

8 servings

In small mixing bowl, combine sauce ingredients. Cover with plastic wrap and chill. In 2-cup measure, combine onion, oil and garlic. Cover with plastic wrap. Microwave at High for 3 to 5 minutes, or until onion is tender, stirring once. Add vinegar, horseradish and red pepper flakes. Mix well. Let cool.

To butterfly roast, make horizontal cut through center of roast to within 1/2 inch of opposite side; do not cut through. Open roast like a book. Place roast in large plastic food-storage bag. Add marinade to bag. Secure bag. Turn to coat. Refrigerate 8 hours or overnight, turning bag occasionally.

Spray cooking grid with nonstick vegetable cooking spray. Prepare grill for medium direct heat. Drain and discard marinade from meat. Place roast on cooking grid. Grill, covered, for 20 to 25 minutes for rare (135°F) to medium (155°F), or to desired doneness, turning once. Let roast stand, tented with foil, for 10 minutes before carving. (Internal temperature will rise 5°F during standing.) Cut roast lengthwise through center to separate into 2 pieces. Carve each piece across grain into thin slices. Top each serving with 2 tablespoons Horseradish Sauce.

Serving suggestion: Serve with steamed fresh broccoli spears.

Per Serving: Calories: 203 • Protein: 25 g. • Carbohydrate: 2 g. • Fat: 10 g.
• Cholesterol: 64 mg. • Sodium: 137 mg.
Exchanges: 3 lean meat, 1/4 vegetable, 3/4 fat

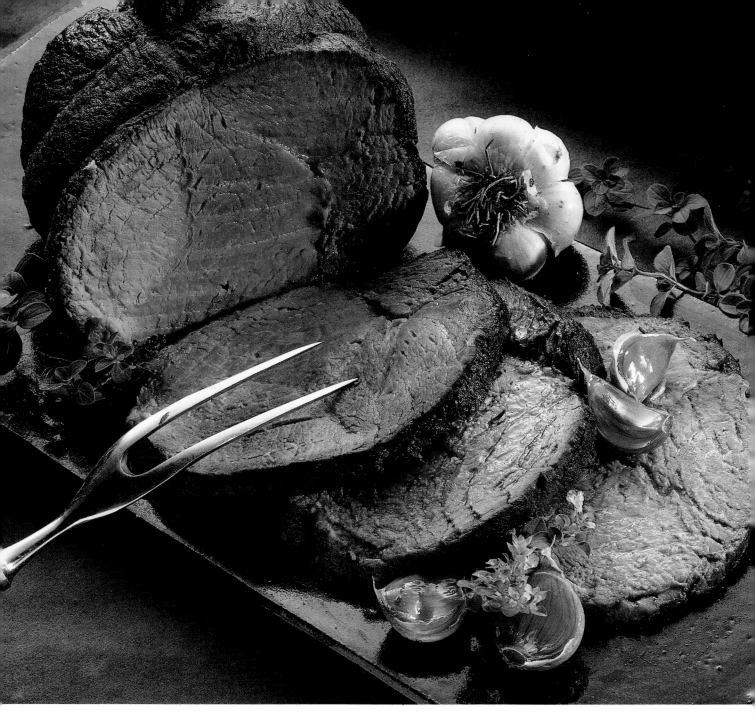

Hickory-smoked Round Tip Roast with Grilled Garlic Spread

Marinade:
1 can (8 oz.) tomato sauce
¼ cup red wine vinegar
2 tablespoons packed brown sugar
2 tablespoons low-sodium Worcestershire sauce
1 clove garlic, minced
¾ teaspoon chili powder
¾ teaspoon freshly ground pepper
1 bay leaf

2- lb. beef round tip roast
4 cups water
2 cups hickory wood smoking chips
2 bulbs garlic (1.5 oz. each)
1 tablespoon olive oil
¼ teaspoon dried oregano leaves

Serving suggestion: Spread insides of kaiser buns with roasted garlic and top with slices of Hickory-smoked Round Tip Roast. Top with barbecue sauce, if desired.

Per Serving: Calories: 189 • Protein: 25 g.
• Carbohydrate: 8 g. • Fat: 6 g.
• Cholesterol: 68 mg. • Sodium: 198 mg.
Exchanges: 3 lean meat, ½ vegetable, ¼ fruit

8 servings

How to Make Hickory-smoked Round Tip Roast with Grilled Garlic Spread

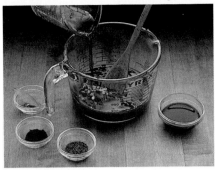

Combine marinade ingredients in 4-cup measure. Cover with plastic wrap. Microwave at High for 4 to 5 minutes, or until marinade begins to boil. Boil for 1 minute. Set aside to cool.

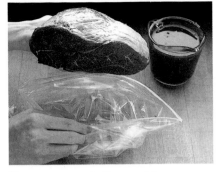

Remove and discard bay leaf. Reserve 1/3 cup marinade. Cover and chill. Place roast in large plastic food-storage bag.

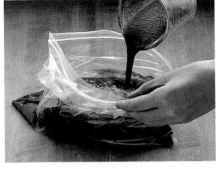

Pour remaining 1 cup marinade over roast. Secure bag. Turn to coat. Refrigerate 8 hours or overnight, turning bag occasionally.

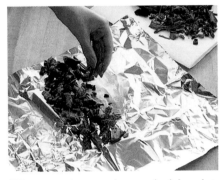

Place water and wood chips in large mixing bowl. Soak chips for 1 hour. Drain on paper towels. Place in center of 16-inch sheet of heavy-duty foil. Bring short edges of foil together and fold down to make log. Set aside.

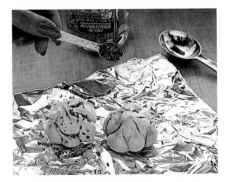

Peel papery layers away from garlic bulbs. Place on 12-inch square piece of heavy-duty aluminum foil. Drizzle with oil. Sprinkle with oregano. Tightly seal foil around garlic bulbs to form packet. Set aside.

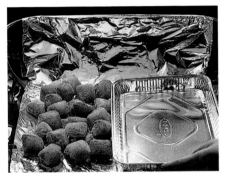

Spray cooking grid with non-stick vegetable cooking spray. Prepare grill for medium indirect heat. Place drip pan on empty side of grill.

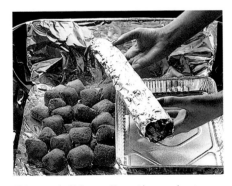

Place foil log directly on hot coals. Drain and discard marinade from meat. Remove meat from bag. Insert meat thermometer in roast. Place roast and garlic packet on cooking grid over drip pan.

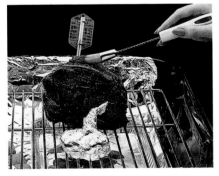

Grill, covered, for 1 hour 15 minutes to 1 hour 30 minutes for rare (135°F) to medium (155°F), or to desired doneness, turning over and basting meat with reserved marinade 3 times. Add additional coals to grill after 1 hour.

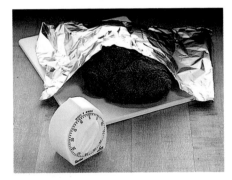

Remove roast and garlic packet from grill. Let roast stand, tented with foil, for 10 minutes. (Internal temperature will rise 5°F during standing.) Carve roast across grain into thin slices. Squeeze garlic from base of each clove and serve as spread.

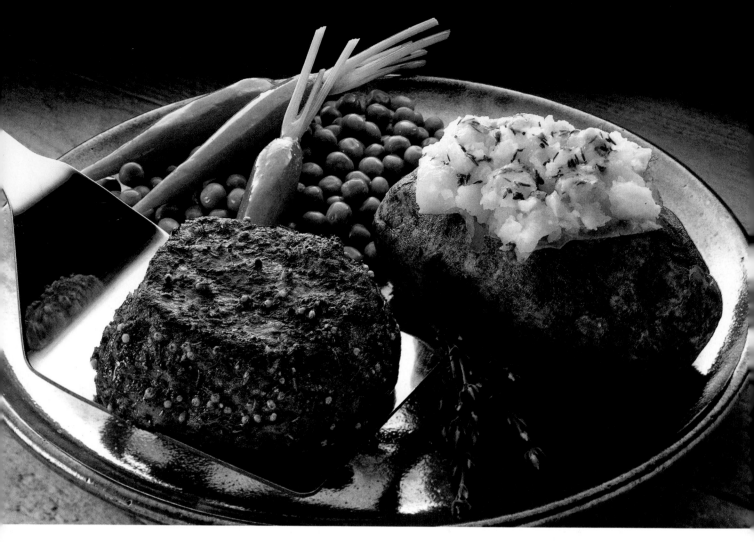

Mustard Steak & Baked Potatoes

Seasoning Mix:

  2 teaspoons dry mustard

1½ teaspoons dried thyme
      leaves

  1 teaspoon mustard seed,
      coarsely crushed

  ¾ teaspoon onion powder

  ½ teaspoon salt

  ½ teaspoon pepper

  1 tablespoon vegetable oil

1- lb. well-trimmed
      boneless beef sirloin
      steak, 1 inch thick

  4 baking potatoes (8 to 10 oz.
      each)

  ¼ cup margarine or butter

1½ teaspoons Dijon mustard

  1 teaspoon dried thyme
      leaves

  ¼ teaspoon salt

  ¼ teaspoon pepper

  ½ cup sliced green onions

4 servings

In small bowl, combine seasoning mix ingredients. Place steak on plate. Spread both sides of steak evenly with seasoning mixture. Cover with plastic wrap. Chill.

Spray cooking grid with nonstick vegetable cooking spray. Prepare grill for medium direct heat. Pierce potatoes with fork. Arrange in circle on paper towel in microwave oven. Microwave at High for 9 to 12 minutes, or until potatoes are hot and yield to slight pressure. Set aside.

In small bowl, microwave margarine at High for 1¼ to 1½ minutes, or until melted. Add mustard, thyme, salt and pepper. Mix well. Place each potato on sheet of heavy-duty foil. Slash each potato lengthwise and then crosswise. Gently press both ends until center pops open. Drizzle 1 tablespoon margarine mixture into each potato. Sprinkle evenly with onions. Wrap foil around each potato and seal.

Arrange potatoes on half of cooking grid. Grill, covered, for 10 minutes. Place steak on remaining half of cooking grid. Grill steak and potatoes, covered, for 12 to 14 minutes, or until meat is desired doneness and potatoes are tender, turning steak over and rearranging potatoes once.

Serving suggestion: Serve with steamed peas and baby carrots.

Per Serving: Calories: 507 • Protein: 32 g. • Carbohydrate: 45 g. • Fat: 22 g.
• Cholesterol: 76 mg. • Sodium: 674 mg.
Exchanges: 3 starch, 3 lean meat, 2½ fat

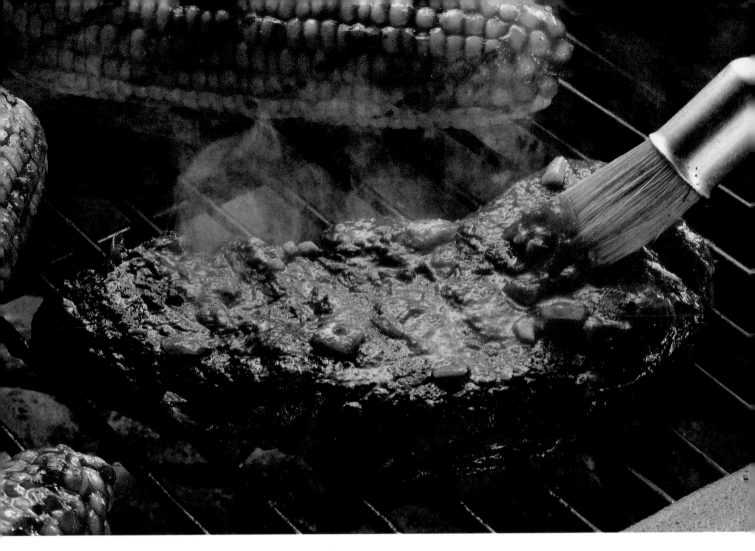

Grilled Chuck Steak with Corn on the Cob

Marinade:

⅓ cup finely chopped onion
2 cloves garlic, minced
1 tablespoon vegetable oil
½ cup red wine vinegar
¼ cup tomato paste
2 tablespoons packed brown
    sugar
1 teaspoon prepared hot
    mustard
2 small dried hot chilies,
    minced
½ teaspoon ground cumin
3 drops red pepper sauce

1-lb. well-trimmed boneless
    beef chuck shoulder steak,
    1 inch thick
4 ears fresh corn on the cob
    (8 oz. each), husked
¼ cup water

4 servings

In small mixing bowl, combine onion, garlic and oil. Microwave at High for 2 to 3 minutes, or until onion is tender, stirring once. Add remaining marinade ingredients. Mix well. Reserve ¼ cup marinade. Cover and chill. Place steak in large plastic food-storage bag. Add remaining marinade. Secure bag. Turn to coat. Chill 4 hours or overnight, turning bag occasionally.

Spray cooking grid with nonstick vegetable cooking spray. Prepare grill for medium direct heat. Arrange corn in 8-inch square baking dish. Add water. Cover with plastic wrap. Microwave at High for 10 to 14 minutes, or until color brightens, rearranging ears once. Set aside.

Drain and discard marinade from meat. Place steak on cooking grid. Grill, covered, for 8 minutes. Turn steak over. Arrange ears of corn around steak. Baste corn with reserved marinade. Grill, covered, for 6 to 8 minutes for rare (140°F) to medium (160°F), or until meat is desired doneness and corn is lightly browned, turning ears 2 or 3 times.

Serving suggestion: Serve with steamed green beans and potato salad.

Per Serving: Calories: 318 • Protein: 32 g. • Carbohydrate: 25 g. • Fat: 11 g.
• Cholesterol: 86 mg. • Sodium: 167 mg.
Exchanges: 1 starch, 3 lean meat, 2 vegetable, ½ fat

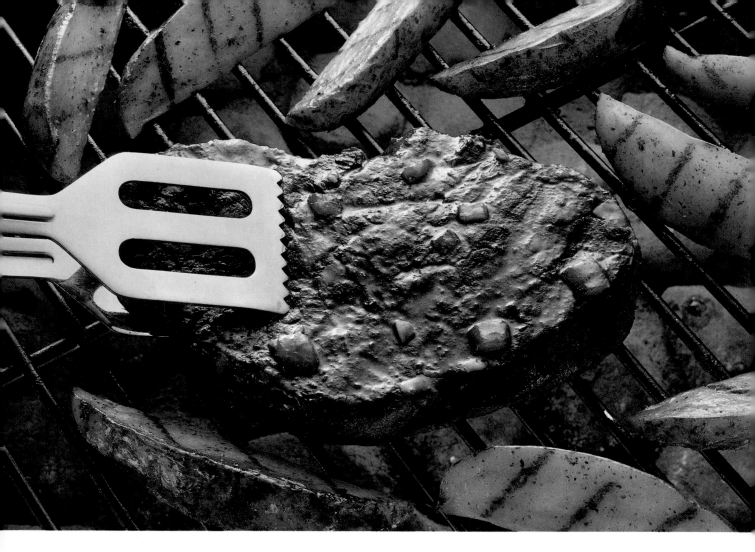

Zesty Beer-marinated Chuck Steak with Ranch-seasoned Steak Fries

Marinade:

½ cup chopped onion
1 tablespoon vegetable oil
1 clove garlic, minced
¾ cup prepared barbecue sauce
½ cup beer
¼ cup packed brown sugar
2 tablespoons lemon juice
2 tablespoons low-sodium Worcestershire sauce
¼ teaspoon cayenne

1 - lb. well-trimmed boneless beef chuck shoulder steak, 1 inch thick
2 baking potatoes (8 to 10 oz. each)
2 tablespoons margarine or butter
1 pkg. (0.4 oz.) ranch dressing mix

4 servings

In small mixing bowl, combine onion, oil and garlic. Cover with plastic wrap. Microwave at High for 2 to 4 minutes, or until onion is tender, stirring once. Add remaining marinade ingredients. Mix well. Place steak in large plastic food-storage bag. Reserve ½ cup marinade. Cover and chill. Add remaining marinade to bag. Secure bag. Turn to coat. Chill 4 hours or overnight, turning bag occasionally.

Spray cooking grid with nonstick vegetable cooking spray. Prepare grill for medium direct heat. Cut each potato lengthwise into 8 wedges. In 10-inch square casserole, microwave margarine at High for 45 seconds to 1 minute, or until melted. Add potatoes, turning to coat. Sprinkle dressing mix evenly over potatoes. Cover. Microwave at High for 10 to 12 minutes, or until potatoes are tender, rearranging once.

Drain and discard marinade from meat. Place steak on cooking grid. Grill, covered, for 8 minutes. Turn steak over. Arrange potato wedges around steak. Baste steak with reserved marinade. Grill, covered, for 6 to 8 minutes for rare (140°F) to medium (160°F), or until meat is desired doneness and potato wedges are lightly browned, turning potatoes 2 or 3 times.

Serving suggestion: Serve with lightly buttered zucchini and yellow summer squash slices.

Per Serving: Calories: 443 • Protein: 32 g. • Carbohydrate: 40 g. • Fat: 16 g. • Cholesterol: 86 mg. • Sodium: 715 mg.
Exchanges: 2 starch, 3 lean meat, 2 vegetable, 1½ fat

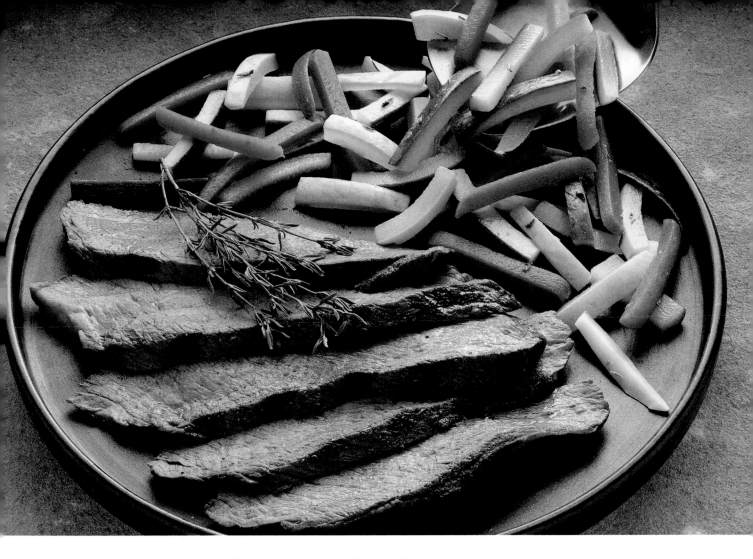

Cajun Crusted Steak with Southern-style Squash

Cajun Seasoning:

2 teaspoons cayenne
1 teaspoon paprika
1/2 teaspoon dried thyme leaves
1/2 teaspoon dried oregano leaves
1 teaspoon salt
3/4 teaspoon pepper
3/4 teaspoon garlic powder
1/2 teaspoon onion powder
2 tablespoons vegetable oil

1- lb. well-trimmed beef top sirloin steak,
   3/4 inch thick
2 medium zucchini squash, cut into 2 × 1/4-inch
   strips
2 medium yellow summer squash, cut into
   2 × 1/4-inch strips
2 medium carrots, cut into
   2 × 1/4-inch strips
2 tablespoons margarine or butter
1/4 teaspoon dried thyme leaves
1/4 teaspoon salt

4 servings

Spray cooking grid with nonstick vegetable cooking spray. Prepare grill for medium direct heat. In small mixing bowl, combine seasoning ingredients. Place steak on plate. Spread both sides of steak evenly with seasoning mixture. Place steak on cooking grid. Grill, covered, for 12 to 14 minutes, or until desired doneness, turning over once.

In 2-quart casserole, combine remaining ingredients. Cover. Microwave at High for 9 to 12 minutes, or until vegetables are tender, stirring twice. Carve sirloin steak into thin slices. Serve with vegetables.

Serving suggestion: Serve with corn bread sticks or muffins.

Per Serving: Calories: 339 • Protein: 29 g.• Carbohydrate: 13 g.
• Fat: 20 g. • Cholesterol: 76 mg. • Sodium: 831 mg.
Exchanges: 3 lean meat, 2½ vegetable, 2 fat

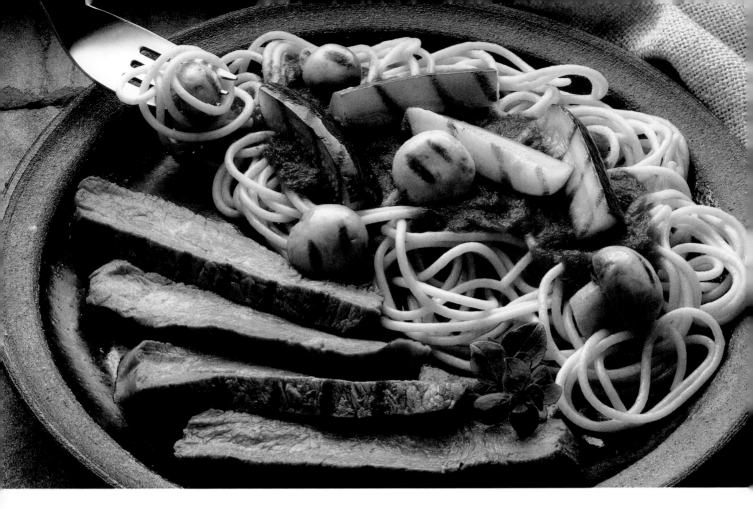

Grilled Italian Steaks & Vegetables with Spaghetti

1 pkg. (7 oz.) uncooked
   spaghetti
2 tablespoons plus 1
   teaspoon olive oil, divided
2 medium zucchini, cut in
   half lengthwise
2 tablespoons water
8 oz. fresh mushrooms
   (2 cups)
2½ teaspoons Italian
   seasoning, divided
1 clove garlic, minced
2 well-trimmed beef top loin
   steaks (8 oz. each), 1 inch
   thick
1 jar (14 oz.) spaghetti sauce

4 servings

Soak three 12-inch wooden skewers in water for ½ hour. Spray cooking grid with nonstick vegetable cooking spray. Prepare grill for medium direct heat. Prepare spaghetti as directed on package. Drain. Toss with 1 teaspoon oil. Cover to keep warm. Set aside. Place zucchini and water in 8-inch square baking dish. Cover with plastic wrap. Microwave at High for 4 to 6 minutes, or until zucchini is tender, re-arranging once. Set aside. Thread mushrooms on skewers. Set aside.

In small bowl, combine remaining 2 tablespoons oil, 1 teaspoon Italian seasoning and the garlic. Brush zucchini and mushrooms with oil mixture. Set aside. Place steaks on plate. Rub both sides of steaks evenly with remaining 1½ teaspoons Italian seasoning. Place steaks on cooking grid. Grill, covered, for 4 minutes. Arrange vege-tables on cooking grid next to steaks. Turn steaks over. Grill, covered, for 8 to 10 minutes, or until meat is desired doneness and vegetables are lightly browned, turning once. Remove meat and vegetables from grill. Slice zucchini into 2 × ½-inch pieces. Cover meat and vegetables to keep warm. Set aside.

Place spaghetti sauce in 4-cup measure. Cover with plastic wrap. Microwave at High for 3 to 4 minutes, or until sauce is hot, stirring once. Place spaghetti on serving platter. Spoon sauce and grilled vegetables over pasta. Carve steaks across grain into thin slices. Serve with pasta.

Serving suggestion: Serve with tossed green salad and garlic toast.

Per Serving: Calories: 570 • Protein: 35 g. • Carbohydrate: 59 g. • Fat: 22 g.
• Cholesterol: 65 mg. • Sodium: 569 mg.
Exchanges: 2 starch, 3 lean meat, 5 vegetable, 2½ fat

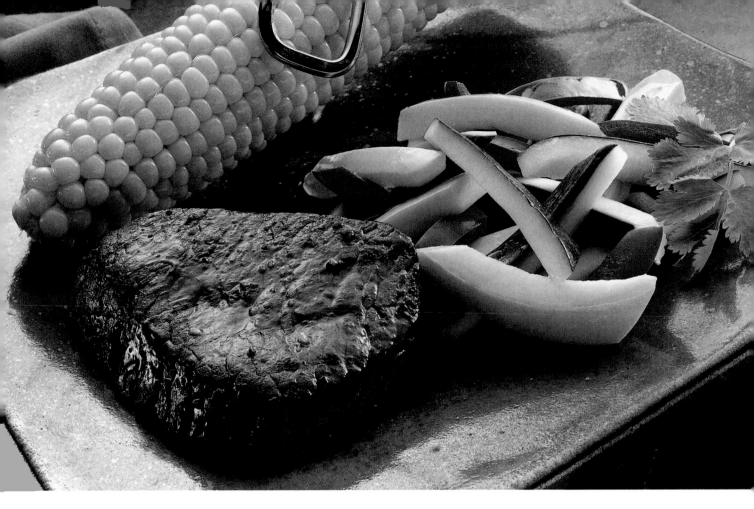

Oriental Barbecued Round Steak with Grilled Corn on the Cob

Marinade:

¼ cup catsup
2 tablespoons reduced-sodium
   soy sauce
2 tablespoons packed brown
   sugar
2 tablespoons red wine
   vinegar
2 cloves garlic, minced
¼ teaspoon pepper

1 - lb. well-trimmed
   boneless beef top round
   steak, ¾ inch thick
4 ears fresh corn on the cob
   (8 oz. each)

4 servings

In small mixing bowl, combine marinade ingredients. Cover with plastic wrap. Microwave at High for 3 to 4 minutes, or until marinade begins to boil, stirring once. Boil for 1 minute. Set aside to cool. Place steak in large plastic food-storage bag. Reserve ¼ cup marinade. Cover and chill. Add remaining marinade to bag. Secure bag. Turn to coat. Chill 4 hours or overnight, turning bag occasionally.

Pull back husks on each ear of corn. Remove and discard silk. Pull husks back up and over ears. Tie tops with string to secure. Soak ears in cold water for ½ hour.

Spray cooking grid with nonstick vegetable cooking spray. Prepare grill for medium direct heat. Drain and discard marinade from meat. Place steak and corn on cooking grid. Grill, covered, for 12 to 14 minutes, or until meat is desired doneness and corn is tender, turning steak over once and basting with reserved marinade and turning corn several times.

Serving suggestion: Serve with steamed fresh julienne yellow summer squash, zucchini and red pepper.

Per Serving: Calories: 275 • Protein: 30 g. • Carbohydrate: 28 g. • Fat: 5 g.
• Cholesterol: 72 mg. • Sodium: 544 mg.
Exchanges: 1⅓ starch, 3 lean meat, ½ fruit

127

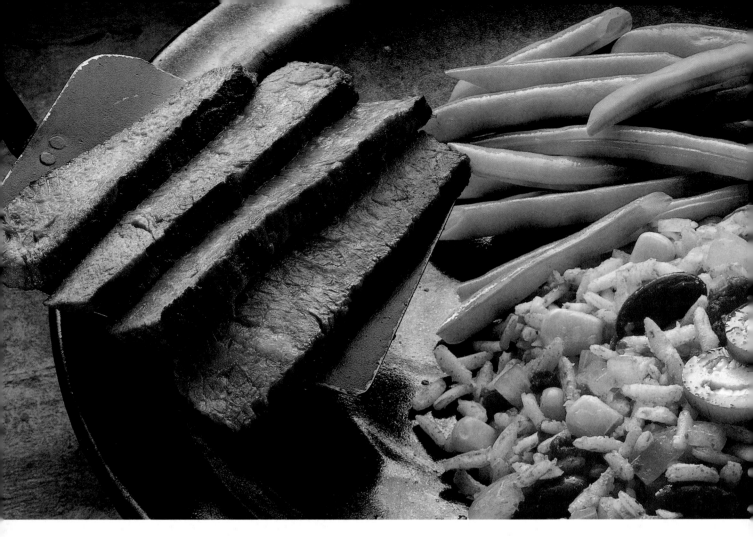

Jalapeño Steak with Southwestern-style Rice

Marinade:
- ⅓ cup salsa
- 2 tablespoons diced canned jalapeño peppers
- 2 teaspoons lemon juice
- ½ teaspoon ground cumin
- ⅛ teaspoon cayenne

- 2 well-trimmed beef top loin steaks (8 oz. each), 1 inch thick
- 1 tablespoon vegetable oil
- ½ cup chopped onion
- 1 clove garlic, minced
- 1¼ cups water
- 1 cup uncooked instant brown rice
- 1 can (8 oz.) diced tomatoes, undrained
- 1 can (8 oz.) kidney beans, rinsed and drained
- ¾ cup frozen corn
- ¼ cup salsa
- ½ teaspoon ground cumin
- ½ teaspoon salt
- ¼ teaspoon chili powder

4 servings

In 1-cup measure, combine marinade ingredients. Place steaks in large plastic food-storage bag. Add marinade. Secure bag. Turn to coat. Chill 2 to 3 hours, turning bag occasionally.

Spray cooking grid with nonstick vegetable cooking spray. Prepare grill for medium direct heat. In 2-quart casserole, combine oil, onion and garlic. Microwave at High for 3 to 5 minutes, or until onion is tender, stirring once. Add remaining ingredients. Mix well. Cover. Microwave at High for 7 to 9 minutes, or until boiling. Microwave at 50% (Medium) for 8 to 12 minutes longer, or until rice is tender and liquid is absorbed. Cover to keep warm. Set aside.

Discard marinade from meat. Place steaks on cooking grid. Grill, covered, for 12 to 14 minutes, or until desired doneness, turning over once. Carve steaks across grain into thin slices. Serve with rice mixture.

Serving suggestion: Serve with steamed whole green beans and tossed salad.

Per Serving: Calories: 385 • Protein: 31 g. • Carbohydrate: 38 g. • Fat: 13 g. • Cholesterol: 65 mg. • Sodium: 690 mg. Exchanges: 2 starch, 3 lean meat, 1½ vegetable, 1 fat

Sun-dried Tomato-stuffed Tenderloin

- 1 cup hot water
- 2 oz. sun-dried tomatoes (about 30 tomatoes)
- 2 tablespoons olive oil, divided
- 3 cloves garlic, minced
- ½ cup snipped fresh basil leaves
- 1-lb. well-trimmed beef tenderloin
- 8 oz. uncooked linguine
- ½ teaspoon salt

4 servings

Place water in 2-cup measure. Microwave at High for 2 to 3 minutes, or until water begins to boil. Add tomatoes. Cover with plastic wrap. Let soak for 15 to 30 minutes, or until tomatoes soften. Drain.

Spray cooking grid with non-stick vegetable cooking spray. Prepare grill for medium direct heat. Cut tomatoes into small pieces. Set aside.

In small mixing bowl, combine 1 tablespoon oil and the garlic. Cover with plastic wrap. Microwave at High for 2 to 2½ minutes, or until garlic is tender, stirring once. Add tomato pieces and basil. Mix well.

Divide tomato mixture in half. Set aside. Make horizontal cut through center of tenderloin to within ½ inch of opposite side; do not cut through. Open tenderloin like a book. Spoon

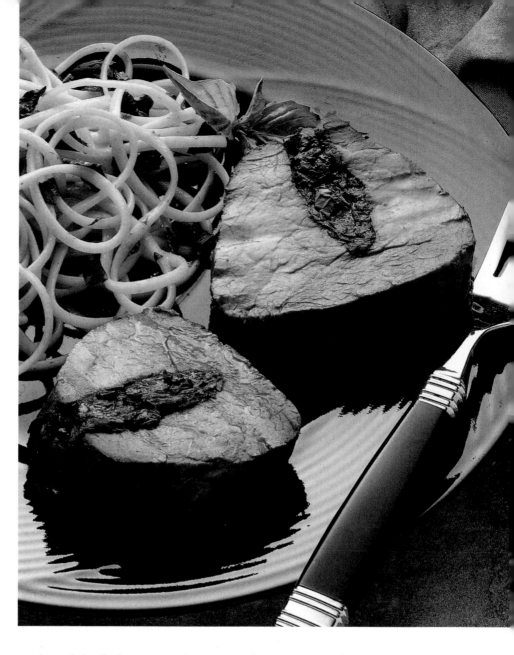

and pack half of tomato mixture down one side of tenderloin. Fold other side of tenderloin over to enclose stuffing.

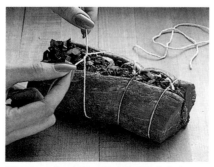

Tie tenderloin at 1½-inch intervals to secure. Place on cooking grid. Grill, covered, for 18 to 24 minutes for rare (135°F) to medium (155°F), or to desired

doneness, turning over once. Remove meat from grill. Cover to keep warm. (Internal temperature will rise 5°F during standing.) Set aside.

Prepare linguine as directed on package. Rinse and drain. Place in large mixing bowl or salad bowl. Add remaining tomato mixture and 1 tablespoon oil and the salt. Toss to combine. Slice tenderloin crosswise into 8 pieces. Serve with linguine.

Serving suggestion: Serve with garlic toast.

Per Serving: Calories: 516 • Protein: 33 g. • Carbohydrate: 55 g. • Fat: 18 g. • Cholesterol: 71 mg. • Sodium: 350 mg. Exchanges: 3 starch, 3 lean meat, 2 vegetable, 2 fat

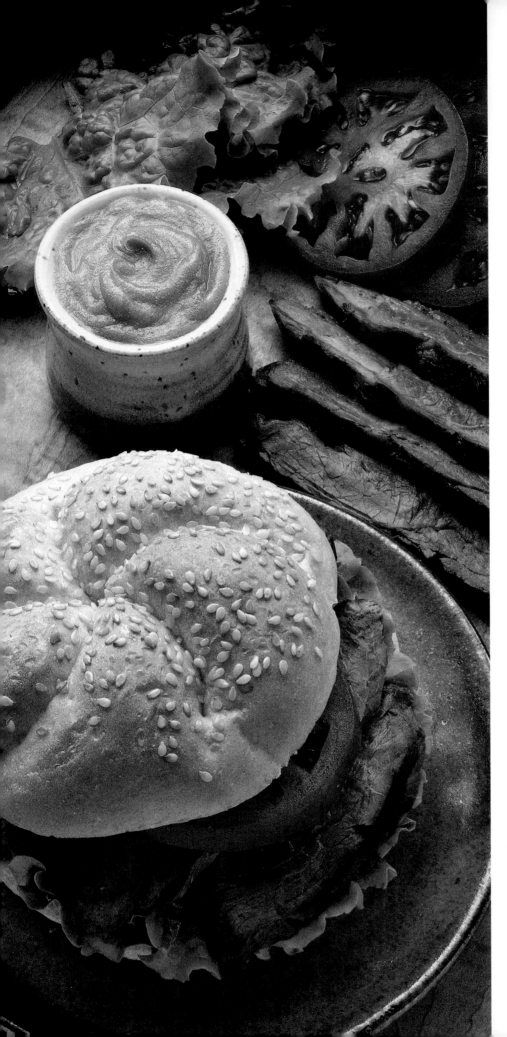

Herbed Flank Steak Sandwiches

Marinade:

⅓ cup chopped onion
1 tablespoon vegetable oil
1 clove garlic, minced
⅓ cup red wine vinegar
1 tablespoon snipped fresh parsley
1 tablespoon snipped fresh oregano leaves
1 tablespoon snipped fresh thyme leaves

1- lb. well-trimmed beef flank steak
4 kaiser rolls, split
Sweet hot mustard
8 slices tomato
Leaf lettuce

4 servings

In 2-cup measure, combine onion, oil and garlic. Cover with plastic wrap. Microwave at High for 2 to 3 minutes, or until onion is tender, stirring once. Add remaining marinade ingredients. Mix well. Set aside to cool.

Score steak with 6 diagonal slashes, about ⅛ inch deep. Place steak in large plastic food-storage bag. Add marinade. Secure bag. Turn to coat. Chill 6 hours or overnight, turning bag occasionally.

Spray cooking grid with nonstick vegetable cooking spray. Prepare grill for medium direct heat. Drain and discard marinade from meat. Place steak on cooking grid. Grill, covered, for 12 to 14 minutes, or until desired doneness, turning over once. Carve steak across grain into thin slices. Spread cut sides of each roll with mustard. Top evenly with steak, tomato and lettuce.

Serving suggestion: Serve with coleslaw.

Per Serving: Calories: 357 • Protein: 28 g.
• Carbohydrate: 32 g. • Fat: 12 g.
• Cholesterol: 59 mg. • Sodium: 385 mg.
Exchanges: 2 starch, 3 lean meat,
¼ vegetable, ½ fat

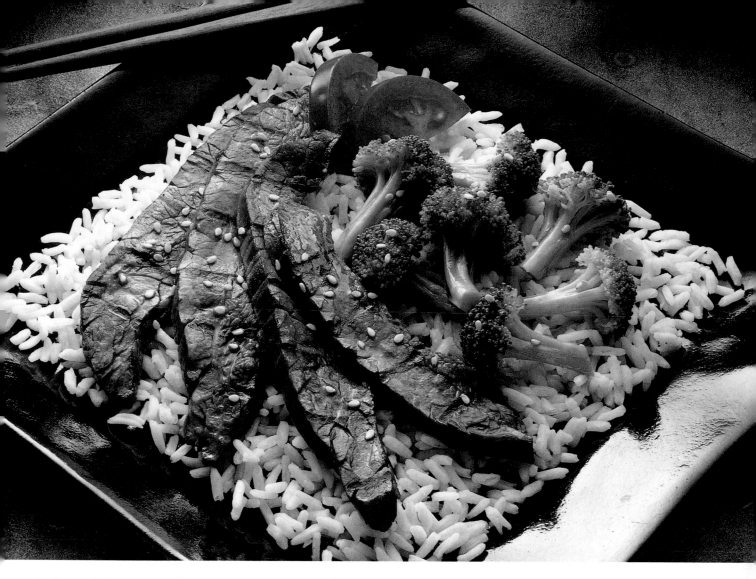

Oriental Sesame Grilled Beef & Broccoli

Marinade:

⅓ cup reduced-sodium soy
    sauce
2 tablespoons sherry
2 tablespoons sesame oil
2 tablespoons packed brown
    sugar
1 tablespoon toasted sesame
    seed
1 teaspoon grated fresh
    gingerroot
2 cloves garlic, minced

1-lb. well-trimmed beef
    flank steak, cut across
    grain into ¼-inch-thick strips
1½ cups uncooked instant rice
1¾ cups water, divided
½ teaspoon salt
3 cups fresh broccoli
    flowerets

4 servings

In 1-cup measure, combine marinade ingredients. Reserve 2 table-spoons marinade. Cover and chill. Place beef strips in large plastic food-storage bag. Add remaining marinade. Secure bag. Turn to coat. Chill 4 hours, turning bag occasionally.

Spray cooking grid with nonstick vegetable cooking spray. Prepare grill for medium direct heat. In 2-quart casserole, combine rice, 1½ cups water and the salt. Cover. Microwave at High for 7 to 8 minutes, or until boiling. Let stand for 5 minutes.

Drain and discard marinade from meat. Place beef strips crosswise on cooking grid. Grill, covered, for 6 to 8 minutes, or until desired doneness, turning over once. Remove meat from grill. Cover to keep warm. Set aside.

In 2-quart casserole, combine broccoli and remaining ¼ cup water. Cover. Microwave at High for 4 to 6 minutes, or until broccoli is tender-crisp, stirring once. Drain. On large serving platter, arrange beef and broccoli over rice. Sprinkle reserved marinade over broccoli.

Serving suggestion: Serve with fresh tomato slices dressed with oil and vinegar.

Per Serving: Calories: 433 • Protein: 30 g. • Carbohydrate: 43 g. • Fat: 15 g.
• Cholesterol: 57 mg. • Sodium: 948 mg.
Exchanges: 2 starch, 3 lean meat, 1 vegetable, ½ fruit, 1 fat

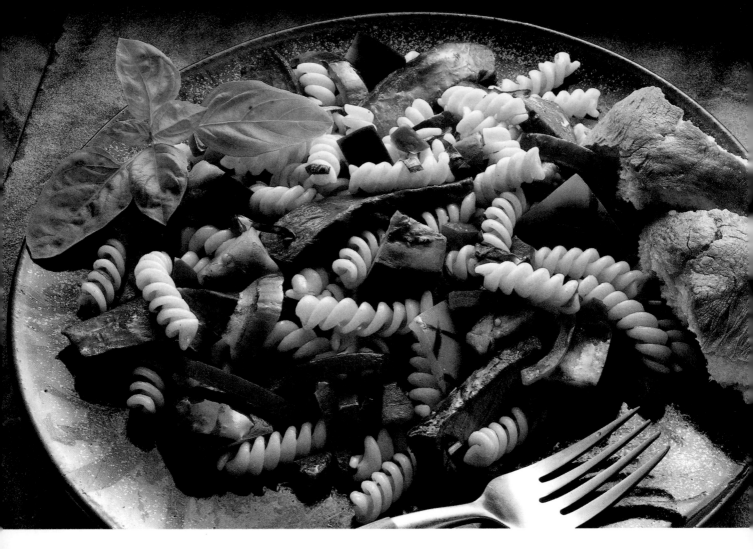

Mediterranean Grilled Salad

6 oz. uncooked rotini
1 medium tomato, seeded
   and chopped
½ cup snipped fresh basil
   leaves
2 tablespoons olive oil
2 tablespoons red wine
   vinegar
1 medium eggplant (1 lb.)
¼ cup water
1- lb. well-trimmed beef top
   sirloin steak, ¾ inch thick
1 medium green pepper,
   seeded and cut into quarters
   lengthwise
½ medium red onion, sliced
   (¼-inch slices)

4 servings

Spray cooking grid with nonstick vegetable cooking spray. Prepare grill for medium direct heat. Prepare rotini as directed on package. Rinse and drain. Place in large mixing bowl or salad bowl. Add tomato and basil. In 1-cup measure, combine oil and vinegar. Add to rotini. Toss to coat. Cover with plastic wrap. Chill.

Cut eggplant lengthwise into ½-inch slices. Place eggplant slices and water in 8-inch square baking dish. Cover with plastic wrap. Microwave at High for 8 to 10 minutes, or until eggplant is almost tender and translucent, rearranging slices twice.

Place steak on cooking grid. Grill, covered, for 4 minutes. Arrange eggplant slices on cooking grid next to steak. Grill, covered, for 3 minutes. Turn steak over. Add green pepper and onion to cooking grid. Grill, covered, for 5 to 7 minutes, or until steak is desired doneness and vegetables are lightly browned and tender, turning vegetables over once during grilling.

Remove steak and vegetables from grill. Carve steak into 2 × ¼-inch strips. Cut eggplant into ½-inch cubes. Cut peppers into 1-inch chunks and onion slices into quarters. Add meat and vegetables to rotini mixture. Toss to combine.

Serving suggestion: Serve with crusty French bread.

Per Serving: Calories: 442 • Protein: 34 g. • Carbohydrate: 45 g. • Fat: 14 g.
• Cholesterol: 76 mg. • Sodium: 69 mg.
Exchanges: 2 starch, 3 lean meat, 3 vegetable, 1 fat

Middle Eastern Skewered Beef with Tabbouleh Salad

Marinade:

¼ cup red wine vinegar
2 tablespoons fresh lemon
   juice
2 tablespoons olive oil
1 tablespoon snipped fresh
   mint leaves
1 clove garlic, minced
1 teaspoon dried oregano
   leaves

1 - lb. well-trimmed boneless
   beef sirloin steak, 1 inch
   thick, cut into 1-inch cubes

Tabbouleh Salad:

1 cup uncooked bulgur
2 cups water
½ cup snipped fresh parsley
¼ cup sliced green onions
2 tablespoons fresh lemon
   juice
2 tablespoons olive oil
2 tablespoons snipped fresh
   mint leaves

3 cups large fresh caulifowerets
¼ cup water
8 cherry tomatoes

4 servings

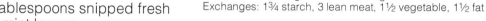

In 1-cup measure, combine marinade ingredients. Place beef cubes in large plastic food-storage bag. Add marinade. Secure bag. Turn to coat. Chill 8 hours or overnight, turning bag occasionally.

Place bulgur in medium mixing bowl. Set aside. Microwave 2 cups water at High for 3 to 4 minutes, or until boiling. Pour over bulgur. Let stand for 15 minutes. Drain excess water. Add remaining salad ingredients to bulgur in bowl. Mix well. Cover with plastic wrap. Chill several hours or overnight.

Soak four 12-inch wooden skewers in water for ½ hour. Spray cooking grid with nonstick vegetable cooking spray. Prepare grill for medium direct heat. In 2-quart casserole, combine cauliflower and water. Cover. Microwave at High for 5 to 7 minutes, or until caulifower is tender, stirring once. Set aside.

Drain and discard marinade from meat. Alternately thread beef cubes, cauliflower and tomatoes on skewers. Place on cooking grid. Grill, covered, for 12 to 14 minutes, or until desired doneness, turning 2 or 3 times. Serve with Tabbouleh Salad.

Serving suggestion: Serve with warm pita loaves.

Per Serving: Calories: 408 • Protein: 32 g. • Carbohydrate: 33 g. • Fat: 17 g.
• Cholesterol: 76 mg. • Sodium: 78 mg.
Exchanges: 1¾ starch, 3 lean meat, 1½ vegetable, 1½ fat

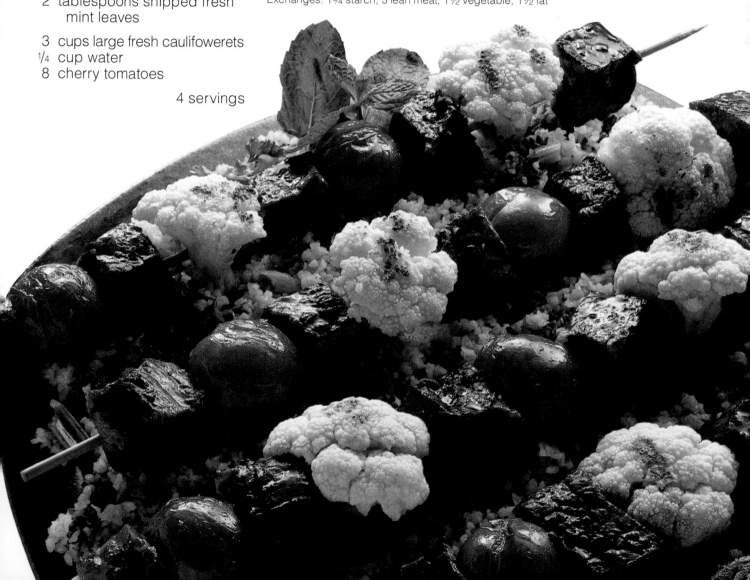

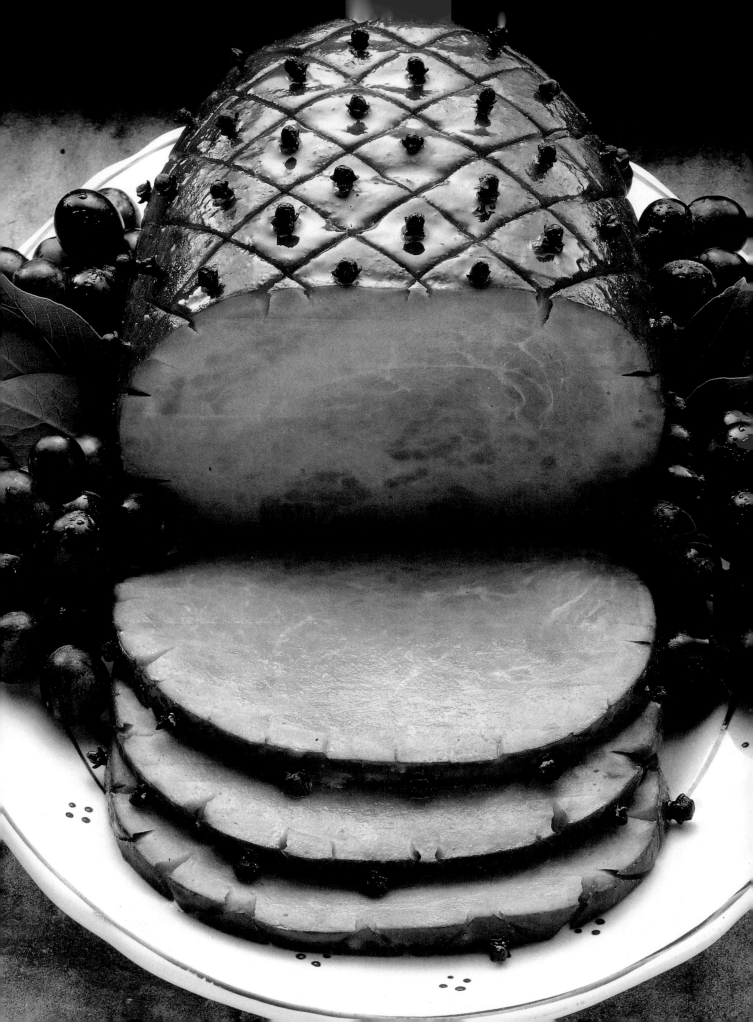

Pork

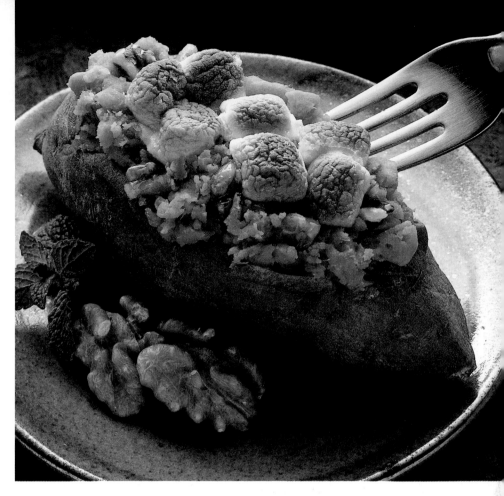

◄ Grilled Mustard-glazed Ham

3 tablespoons margarine or butter
¼ cup packed brown sugar
2 tablespoons Dijon mustard
3-lb. fully cooked boneless ham
Whole cloves

12 servings

In small mixing bowl, microwave margarine at High for 1 to 1¼ minutes, or until melted. Add sugar and mustard. Mix well. Set glaze aside.

Spray cooking grid with non-stick vegetable cooking spray. Prepare grill for medium indirect heat. Place drip pan on empty side of grill.

Score ham in 1-inch diamond pattern, cutting ¼ inch deep. Insert 1 clove in center of each diamond. Cover cut surface of ham with foil. Insert meat thermometer. Place ham on cooking grid over drip pan. Grill, covered, for 1 hour to 1 hour 10 minutes, or until internal temperature registers 135°F, rotating ham twice and brushing with glaze during last 10 minutes of grilling time. Remove ham from grill. Let stand, tented with foil, for 10 minutes. (Internal temperature will rise 5°F during standing.)

Serving suggestion: Serve with Candied Sweet Potatoes, right, and steamed whole green and wax beans or asparagus spears.

Note: Tightly wrap and refrigerate any leftover ham up to 10 days.

Per Serving: Calories: 158 • Protein: 18 g. • Carbohydrate: 5 g. • Fat: 7 g. • Cholesterol: 45 mg. • Sodium: 1106 mg. Exchanges: 3 lean meat, ⅓ fruit

Candied Sweet Potatoes ▲

4 sweet potatoes (8 to 10 oz. each)
1 tablespoon margarine or butter
2 tablespoons packed brown sugar
2 tablespoons chopped walnuts
¼ teaspoon ground cinnamon
¼ cup miniature marshmallows

4 servings

Prepare grill for medium direct heat. Pierce potatoes with fork. Arrange in circle on paper towel in microwave oven. Microwave at High for 9 to 12 minutes, or until potatoes are hot and yield to slight pressure. Set aside. In small mixing bowl, microwave margarine at High for 45 seconds to 1 minute, or until melted. Add sugar, walnuts and cinnamon. Mix well.

Place each potato on sheet of heavy-duty foil. Slash each potato lengthwise and then crosswise. Gently press both ends until center pops open. Spoon about 1 tablespoon sugar mixture into each potato. Wrap foil around potatoes to seal. Place potatoes on cooking grid. Grill, covered, for 15 to 17 minutes, or until tender, rearranging once. Remove potatoes from grill. Open foil and roll down around potatoes, exposing tops. Sprinkle 1 tablespoon marshmallows over top of each potato. Place potatoes on grill. Grill, covered, for 2 to 3 minutes, or until marshmallows are puffed and golden brown.

Serving suggestion: Serve with Grilled Mustard-glazed Ham, left.

Per Serving: Calories: 280 • Protein: 4 g. • Carbohydrate: 55 g. • Fat: 6 g. • Cholesterol: 0 • Sodium: 61 mg. Exchanges: 3 starch, ½ fruit, 1 fat

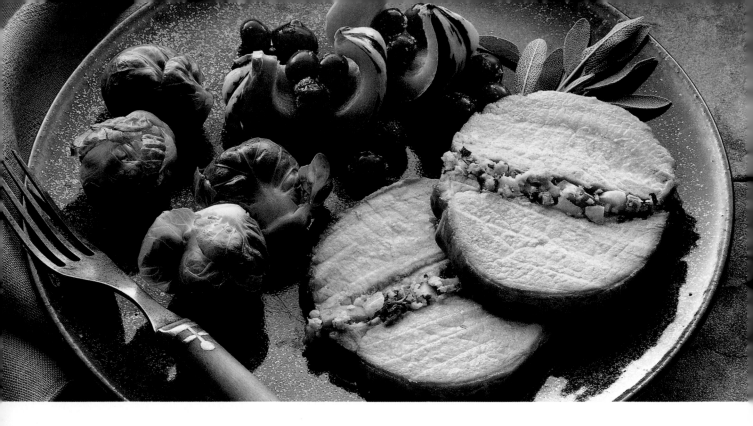

Apple-Sage Stuffed Pork Loin Roast

1/4 cup apple jelly
1 tablespoon packed brown sugar
1 1/2 teaspoons Dijon mustard
1 large apple, cored and chopped (1 cup)
1/2 cup chopped celery
1/2 cup chopped onion
2 tablespoons margarine or butter
1/2 cup unseasoned dry bread crumbs
1/4 cup snipped fresh parsley
2 tablespoons snipped fresh sage leaves
3-lb. well-trimmed boneless pork double loin roast

12 servings

Serving suggestion: Serve with Brussels sprouts and squash.

Note: Tightly wrap and refrigerate any leftover pork up to 4 days, or package in freezer containers or bags and freeze 3 to 4 months.

Per Serving: Calories: 231 • Protein: 25 g. • Carbohydrate: 12 g. • Fat: 11 g. • Cholesterol: 67 mg. • Sodium: 133 mg. Exchanges: 3 lean meat, 1 vegetable, 1/2 fruit, 1/2 fat

In 1-cup measure, combine jelly, sugar and mustard. Microwave at High for 2 to 2 1/2 minutes, or until jelly is melted, stirring once. Cover with plastic wrap. Set glaze aside. In 2-quart casserole, combine apple, celery, onion and margarine. Cover. Microwave at High for 5 to 8 minutes, or until apple is tender, stirring once. Add bread crumbs, parsley and sage. Mix well.

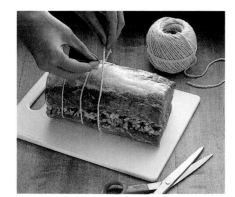

Untie pork roast. Separate the two pieces of loin. Spoon and pack stuffing mixture on top of one pork loin piece. Place remaining loin piece over stuffing. Tie at 1 1/2-inch intervals to secure.

Spray cooking grid with non-stick vegetable cooking spray. Prepare grill for medium indirect heat. Place roast in 8-inch square baking dish. Cover with wax paper or microwave cooking paper. Microwave at 70% (Medium High) for 10 to 15 minutes, or just until exterior is no longer pink, turning roast over after half the cooking time.

Place drip pan on empty side of grill. Insert meat thermometer. Place roast on cooking grid over drip pan. Grill, covered, for 1 hour to 1 hour 30 minutes, or until internal temperature registers 155°F and juices run clear, turning roast over 4 times during grilling and basting with glaze during last 15 minutes of grilling time. Add additional coals to grill after 1 hour. Remove roast from grill. Let stand, tented with foil, for 10 minutes. (Internal temperature will rise 5°F during standing.)

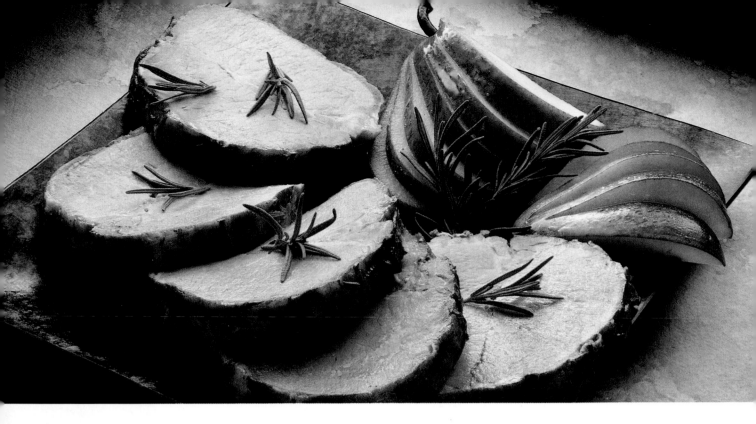

Chardonnay Pork Roast & Pears

Marinade:

- ½ cup chardonnay or other dry white wine
- 2 tablespoons white wine vinegar
- 2 tablespoons vegetable oil
- 1 tablespoon chopped fresh rosemary leaves
- 2 cloves garlic, minced

- 3-lb. well-trimmed boneless pork double loin roast
- 4 medium pears (8 oz. each)
- ¼ cup water
- ½ cup chardonnay or other dry white wine
- ¼ cup packed brown sugar
- 1 teaspoon chopped fresh rosemary leaves

12 servings

Serving suggestion: Serve with steamed whole baby carrots and tossed green salad.

Note: Tightly wrap and refrigerate any leftover pork up to 4 days, or package in freezer containers or bags and freeze 3 to 4 months.

Per Serving: Calories: 252 • Protein: 27 g. • Carbohydrate: 15 g. • Fat: 8 g. • Cholesterol: 68 mg. • Sodium: 57 mg. Exchanges: 3 lean meat, 1 fruit

In 1-cup measure, combine marinade ingredients. Untie pork roast. Separate the two pieces of loin. Place loin pieces in large plastic food-storage bag. Add marinade. Secure bag. Turn to coat. Chill 1 to 2 hours, turning bag once or twice.

Core and cut each pear in half lengthwise. Arrange pear halves cut-sides-up in 10-inch square casserole. Pour water over pear halves. Cover. Microwave at High for 5 to 7 minutes, or until fruit is tender-crisp, rearranging pieces once. Drain. Slice each pear half lengthwise at ¼-inch intervals, starting ½ inch from stem end. Pear halves should remain intact. Return pear halves to same casserole. In 1-cup measure, combine chardonnay, sugar and rosemary. Pour over pears. Cover and chill.

Spray cooking grid with nonstick vegetable cooking spray. Prepare grill for medium indirect heat. Drain and discard marinade from meat. Remove meat from bag. Place loin pieces together. Tie at 1½-inch intervals to secure. Place roast in 8-inch square baking dish. Cover with wax paper or microwave cooking paper. Microwave at 70% (Medium High) for 10 to 15 minutes, or just until exterior is no longer pink, turning roast over after half the cooking time. Place drip pan on empty side of grill. Insert meat thermometer. Place roast on cooking grid over drip pan. Grill, covered, for 1 hour to 1 hour 30 minutes, or until internal temperature registers 155°F and juices run clear, turning roast over 4 times during grilling. Add additional coals to grill after 1 hour. Remove roast from grill. Let stand, tented with foil, for 10 minutes. (Internal temperature will rise 5°F during standing.)

Arrange pear halves over direct heat side of cooking grid. Grill, covered, for 8 to 10 minutes, or until pears are lightly browned and tender, turning over once and basting with chardonnay mixture twice. Carve roast across grain into thin slices. Arrange on serving platter. Garnish with pear halves.

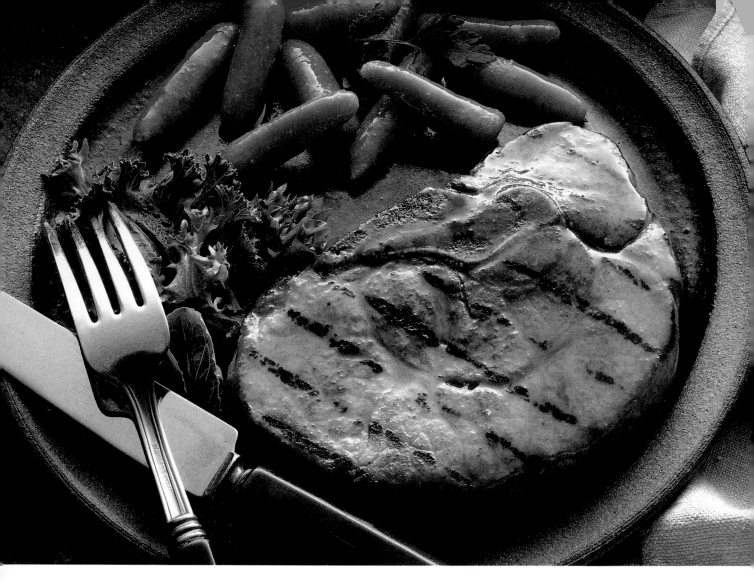

Honey-Mustard Chops & Carrots

5 tablespoons honey
2 tablespoons packed brown
   sugar
2 tablespoons Dijon mustard
1 pkg. (14 oz.) frozen whole
   baby carrots
2 tablespoons water
4 well-trimmed bone-in pork
   sirloin chops (6 oz. each),
   3/4 inch thick

4 servings

In 2-cup measure, combine honey, sugar and mustard. Microwave at High for 2 to 2½ minutes, or until sugar is melted, stirring once. Set glaze aside. In 2-quart casserole, combine carrots and water. Cover. Microwave at High for 7 to 9 minutes, or until hot, stirring once. Drain. Add 3 tablespoons glaze to carrots. Toss to coat. Cover. Set aside.

Spray cooking grid with nonstick vegetable cooking spray. Prepare grill for medium direct heat. In 10-inch square casserole, arrange chops with meaty portions toward outside. Cover with wax paper or microwave cooking paper. Microwave at 70% (Medium High) for 6 to 8 minutes, or just until edges of chops are no longer pink, turning over once.

Place chops on cooking grid. Grill, covered, for 8 to 10 minutes, or just until meat is no longer pink, turning and basting with remaining glaze 3 or 4 times. Arrange pork chops on serving platter. Cover to keep warm. Microwave carrots at High for 1 to 2 minutes, or until hot.

Serving suggestion: Serve with tossed green salad.

Per Serving: Calories: 322 • Protein: 26 g. • Carbohydrate: 39 g. • Fat: 10 g.
• Cholesterol: 72 mg. • Sodium: 340 mg.
Exchanges: 3 lean meat, 1¾ vegetable, 2 fruit

138

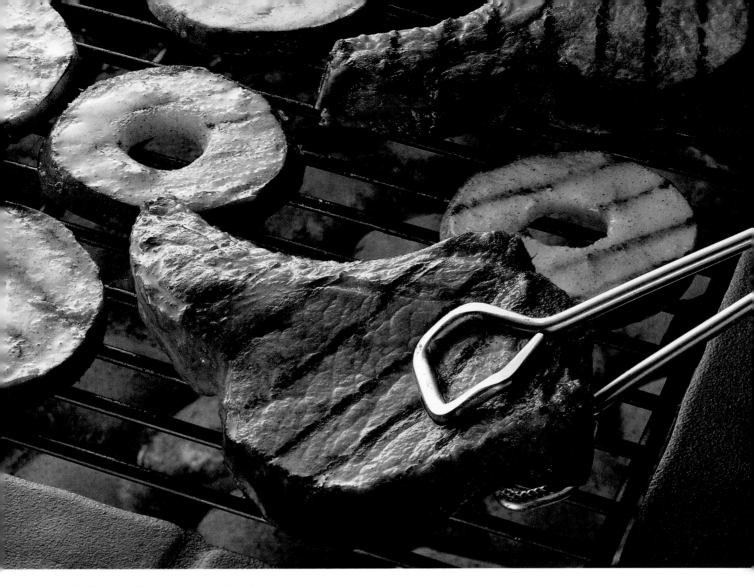

Grilled Pork Chops with Apples

1 Granny Smith apple, cored
   and sliced crosswise into
   1/4-inch slices
1 Rome apple, cored and
   sliced crosswise into
   1/4-inch slices
1 tablespoon water
1 tablespoon lemon juice
3 tablespoons margarine or
   butter
1/4 cup packed brown sugar
1/2 teaspoon ground allspice
4 well-trimmed bone-in pork
   rib or loin chops (8 oz. each),
   1 inch thick
2 tablespoons chopped
   walnuts (optional)

4 servings

Arrange apple slices in 8-inch square baking dish. Sprinkle with water and juice. Cover with plastic wrap. Microwave at High for 4 to 6 minutes, or until apples are tender, rearranging slices once. Drain. Set aside. In small bowl, microwave margarine at High for 1 to 1 1/4 minutes, or until melted. Add sugar and allspice. Mix well. Pour over apples. Set aside.

Spray cooking grid with nonstick vegetable cooking spray. Prepare grill for medium direct heat. In 8-inch square baking dish, arrange pork chops with meaty portions toward outside. Cover with wax paper or microwave cooking paper. Microwave at 70% (Medium High) for 6 to 8 minutes, or just until edges of chops are no longer pink, turning over once.

Place chops on cooking grid. Grill, covered, for 8 to 10 minutes, or just until meat is no longer pink, turning once. Arrange apple slices next to chops on cooking grid during last 4 to 5 minutes of cooking time. Grill until lightly browned, turning over once. Arrange chops and apples on serving platter. Sprinkle with walnuts.

Serving suggestion: Serve with spinach salad and saffron rice.

Per Serving: Calories: 379 • Protein: 26 g. • Carbohydrate: 30 g. • Fat: 17 g.
• Cholesterol: 69 mg. • Sodium: 161 mg.
Exchanges: 3 lean meat, 2 fruit, 1 3/4 fat

Sweet & Sour Pork Kabobs with Pineapple Rice ▶

Marinade:

¼ cup reduced-sodium soy sauce

¼ cup rice wine vinegar

¼ cup packed brown sugar

2 tablespoons vegetable oil

½ teaspoon ground ginger

1 clove garlic, minced

1-lb. well-trimmed boneless pork loin roast, cut into 1-inch cubes

1 cup uncooked long-grain white rice

2 cups water

½ teaspoon salt

1 can (8 oz.) pineapple tidbits, drained (reserve juice)

3 green onions, sliced diagonally into ½-inch lengths (⅓ cup)

8 oz. fresh mushrooms, stems removed (2 cups)

1 medium red pepper, cut into 12 chunks

1 medium green pepper, cut into 12 chunks

Sauce:

¼ cup packed brown sugar

1 tablespoon cornstarch

½ cup reserved pineapple juice

¼ cup vinegar

1 teaspoon reduced-sodium soy sauce

4 servings

Serving suggestion: Serve with hot-and-sour or egg drop soup.

Per Serving: Calories: 556 • Protein: 31 g. • Carbohydrate: 81 g. • Fat: 14 g. • Cholesterol: 67 mg. • Sodium: 826 mg. Exchanges: 2 starch, 3 lean meat, 2 vegetable, 2¾ fruit, 1 fat

How to Make Sweet & Sour Pork Kabobs with Pineapple Rice

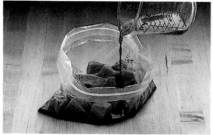

Combine marinade ingredients in 2-cup measure. Reserve ¼ cup marinade. Cover and chill. Place pork in large plastic food-storage bag. Add remaining marinade. Secure bag. Turn to coat. Chill 1 to 2 hours, turning bag occasionally.

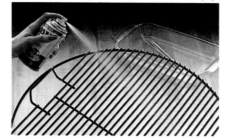

Soak four 12-inch wooden skewers in water for ½ hour. Spray cooking grid with non-stick vegetable cooking spray. Prepare the grill for medium direct heat.

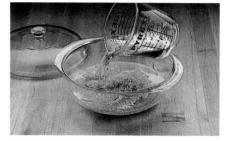

Combine rice, water and salt in 2-quart casserole. Cover. Microwave at High for 5 minutes. Microwave at 50% (Medium) for 15 to 20 minutes longer, or until rice is tender and liquid is absorbed.

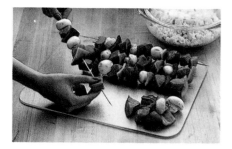

Stir in pineapple and onions. Cover to keep warm. Set aside. Drain and discard marinade from meat. Alternately thread pork cubes, mushrooms and pepper chunks onto skewers. Place kabobs on cooking grid.

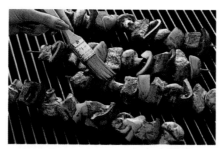

Grill, covered, for 12 to 15 minutes, or until meat is firm and no longer pink, turning kabobs over and basting with reserved marinade 2 or 3 times. Remove kabobs from grill. Cover to keep warm. Set aside.

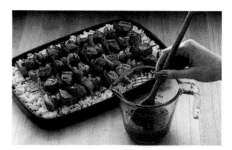

Combine sugar and cornstarch in 2-cup measure. Blend in juice, vinegar and soy sauce. Microwave at High for 3 to 4 minutes, or until thickened and translucent, stirring twice. On large serving platter, arrange kabobs over rice. Spoon sauce over kabobs.

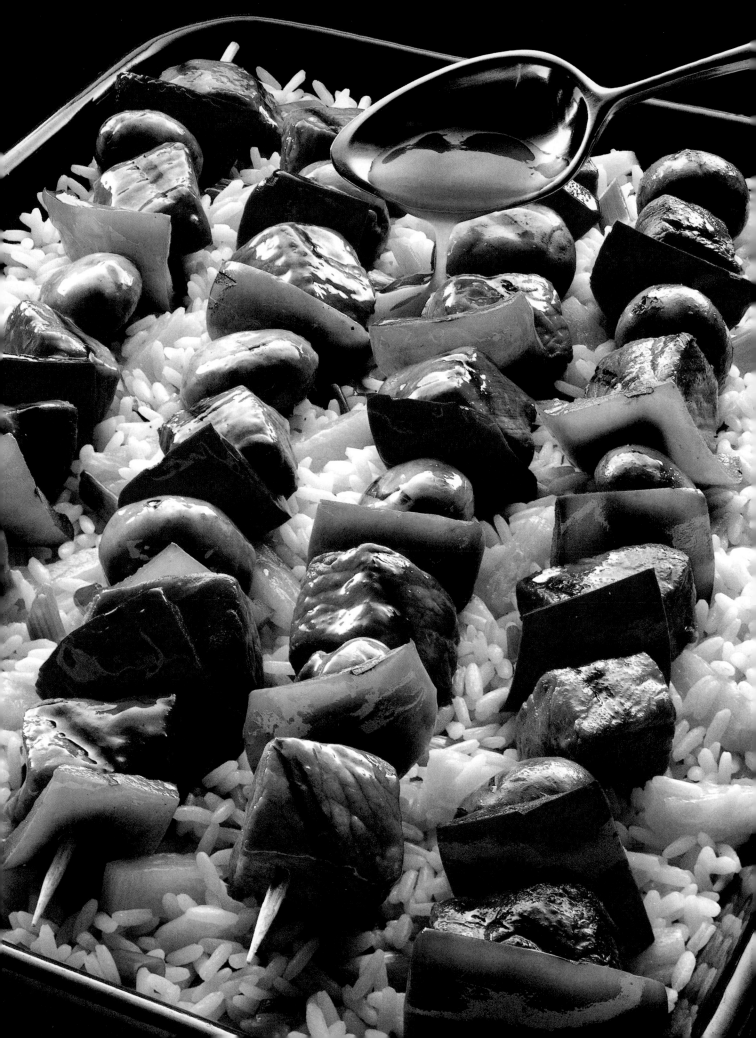

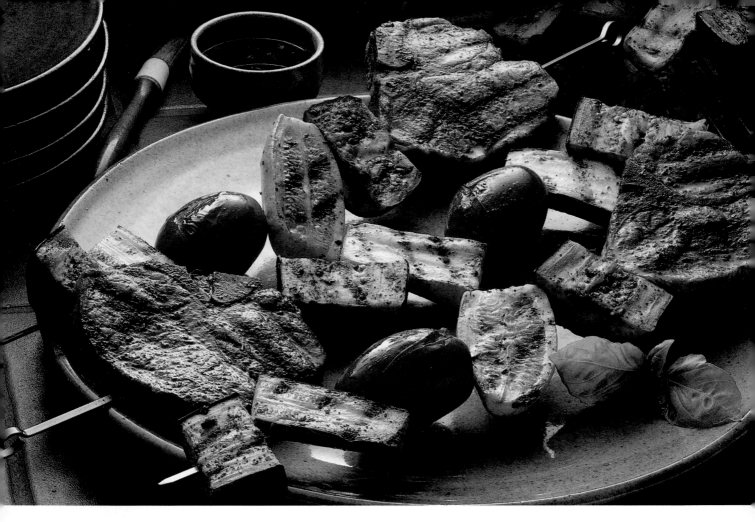

Skewered Pork Chops & Vegetables

Seasoning Blend:

½ teaspoon seasoned salt
½ teaspoon bouquet garni
    seasoning
¼ teaspoon paprika
¼ teaspoon onion powder
¼ teaspoon pepper

3 tablespoons olive oil
2 tablespoons snipped fresh
    basil leaves
2 teaspoons lemon juice
1 clove garlic, minced
1 medium eggplant (1 lb.),
    cut in half lengthwise, then
    crosswise into 1-inch slices
2 medium yellow or green
    zucchini, cut in half
    lengthwise, then crosswise
    into 2-inch lengths
¼ cup water
4 well-trimmed bone-in pork
    center loin or rib chops
    (8 oz. each), 1 inch thick
4 Roma tomatoes

4 servings

In small bowl, combine seasoning blend ingredients. Remove ½ teaspoon of seasoning blend and place in 1-cup measure. Add oil, basil, juice and garlic. Mix well. Set aside seasoning blend and oil mixture.

Spray cooking grid with nonstick vegetable cooking spray. Prepare grill for medium direct heat. Place eggplant and zucchini in 10-inch square casserole. Add water. Cover. Microwave at High for 10 to 12 minutes, or until vegetables are tender, rearranging pieces twice. Set aside.

Rub both sides of each chop evenly with seasoning blend. Arrange chops in 8-inch square baking dish, with meaty portions toward outside. Cover with wax paper or microwave cooking paper. Microwave at 70% (Medium High) for 6 to 8 minutes, or just until edges of chops are no longer pink, turning over once.

Thread pork chop, 2 pieces each of eggplant and zucchini and 1 tomato on each of four 16-inch metal skewers. Brush oil mixture evenly on vegetables. Place skewers on cooking grid. Grill, covered, for 8 to 10 minutes, or just until meat is no longer pink, turning over once.

Serving suggestion: Serve with hot cooked rice.

Per Serving: Calories: 327 • Protein: 29 g. • Carbohydrate: 14 g. • Fat: 18 g.
• Cholesterol: 70 mg. • Sodium: 219 mg.
Exchanges: 3 lean meat, 3 vegetable, 2 fat

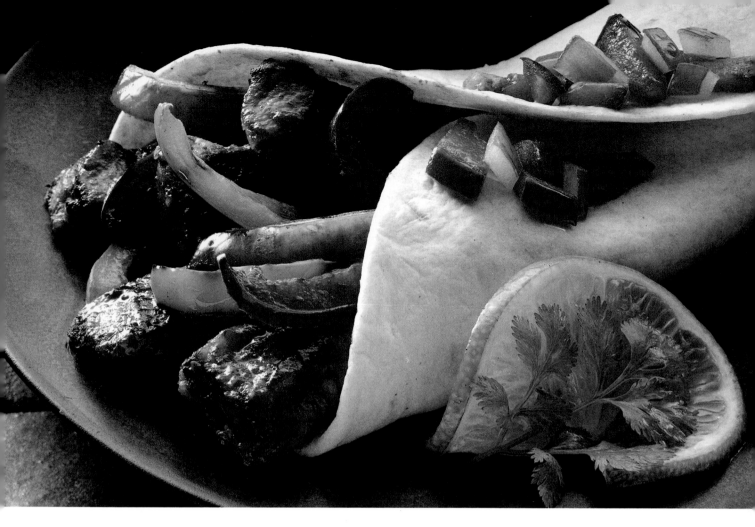

Barbecue Pork Fajitas

4 well-trimmed boneless pork
     top loin chops (4 oz. each),
     cut into 4 × ½-inch-thick
     strips
¼ cup prepared barbecue
     sauce
1 medium green pepper, cut
     into ¼-inch strips
1 medium red pepper, cut
     into ¼-inch strips
2 tablespoons vegetable oil,
     divided
1 medium red onion, sliced
     (¼-inch slices)
4 flour tortillas (8-inch)

4 servings

In medium mixing bowl, combine pork strips and barbecue sauce. Set aside. In another medium mixing bowl, combine pepper strips and 1 tablespoon oil. Toss to coat. Set aside. Place onion slices on plate. Brush both sides with remaining 1 tablespoon oil. Set aside.

Spray cooking grid with nonstick vegetable cooking spray. Prepare grill for medium direct heat. Place pork strips crosswise on cooking grid. Grill for 6 to 8 minutes, or until meat is slightly firm and no longer pink, turning over once. Remove meat from grill. Cover to keep warm. Set aside. Arrange pepper strips and onion slices crosswise on cooking grid. Grill for 5 to 7 minutes, or until tender. Remove vegetables from cooking grid. Cut onion slices in half. Set vegetables aside.

Place tortillas between 2 dampened paper towels. Microwave at High for 45 seconds to 1 minute, or just until tortillas are warm to the touch. Spoon pork, peppers and onions evenly over tortillas. Fold each tortilla up from bottom. Fold in sides and secure with wooden pick, leaving top open. Top with light sour cream and salsa and garnish with fresh cilantro, if desired.

Serving suggestion: Serve with corn on the cob and tossed green salad.

Per Serving: Calories: 413 • Protein: 32 g. • Carbohydrate: 37 g. • Fat: 15 g.
• Cholesterol: 68 mg. • Sodium: 402 mg.
Exchanges: 1½ starch, 3 lean meat, 3 vegetable, 1 fat

143

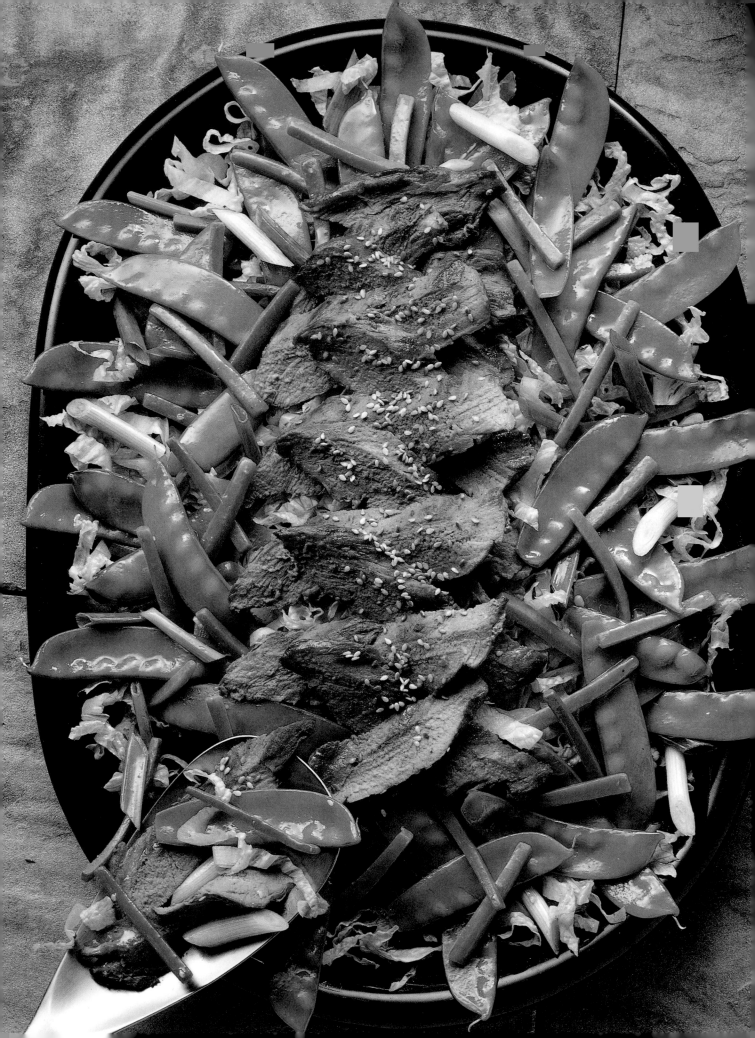

◄ Warm Sesame Pork Salad

Dressing:

- 3 tablespoons vegetable oil
- 2 tablespoons rice wine vinegar
- 1 teaspoon reduced-sodium soy sauce
- 1¼ teaspoons sugar
- ½ teaspoon ground ginger

Marinade:

- ⅓ cup reduced-sodium soy sauce
- 3 tablespoons rice wine vinegar
- 2 tablespoons sesame oil
- 2 tablespoons packed brown sugar
- 1 teaspoon ground ginger
- ½ teaspoon garlic powder

- 1 well-trimmed pork tenderloin (approx. 1 lb.)
- 2 cups fresh snow pea pods
- 1 cup carrot strips (2 × ¼-inch strips)
- 3 tablespoons water
- 3 cups shredded romaine lettuce
- 4 green onions, sliced diagonally into 1-inch lengths (½ cup)
- 2 teaspoons toasted sesame seed

4 servings

In 1-cup measure, combine dressing ingredients. Cover with plastic wrap. Chill. In small mixing bowl, combine marinade ingredients. Set aside. Make horizontal cut through center of pork tenderloin to within ½ inch of opposite side; do not cut through. Open tenderloin like a book. Pound to an even ½-inch thickness. Place in large plastic food-storage bag. Add marinade. Secure bag. Turn to coat. Chill 1 to 2 hours, turning bag twice.

In 2-quart casserole, place pea pods, carrots and water. Cover. Microwave at High for 2 to 3 minutes, or until carrots are tender-crisp and pea pods brighten in color, stirring once. Rinse with cold water. Drain. On large serving platter, arrange lettuce, pea pods, carrots and onions. Set aside.

Spray cooking grid with nonstick vegetable cooking spray. Prepare grill for medium direct heat. Drain and discard marinade from meat. Place tenderloin on cooking grid. Grill, covered, for 7 to 10 minutes, or until internal temperature registers 160°F and juices run clear. Carve pork diagonally into thin slices and arrange in center of platter. Pour dressing over salad and sprinkle with toasted sesame seed.

Serving suggestion: Serve with fortune cookies.

Per Serving: Calories: 358 • Protein: 30 g. • Carbohydrate: 17 g. • Fat: 20 g. • Cholesterol: 80 mg. • Sodium: 531 mg.
Exchanges: 3 lean meat, 2½ vegetable, ⅓ fruit, 2¼ fat

Grilled Pork & Tropical Fruit Salad

- ½ cup guava or passion fruit jelly
- ¼ cup unsweetened pineapple juice or orange juice
- 1 tablespoon lemon juice
- 2 bananas, cut into 2-inch lengths
- 1 papaya, peeled and cut into 1½-inch cubes
- 1 mango, peeled and cut into 1½-inch cubes
- ½ medium pineapple (1½ to 2 lb.), peeled, cored and cut into 1½-inch cubes
- 1 well-trimmed pork tenderloin (approx. 1 lb.)
- 3 cups torn romaine lettuce

Dressing:

- ⅓ cup fresh lime juice
- 2 tablespoons honey
- 2 tablespoons vegetable oil

4 servings

Soak four 12-inch wooden skewers in water for ½ hour. In 2-cup measure, combine jelly, pineapple juice and lemon juice. Microwave at High for 3 to 4 minutes, or until jelly is melted, stirring twice. Set aside.

Alternate fruits evenly on skewers. Arrange in even layer in 13 × 9-inch baking dish. Pour jelly mixture over kabobs, turning to coat fruit. Set aside. Spray cooking grid with nonstick vegetable cooking spray. Prepare grill for medium direct heat.

Place pork on cooking grid. Grill, covered, for 20 to 25 minutes, or until internal temperature registers 155°F and juices run clear. Remove meat from grill. Let stand, tented with foil, for 10 minutes. (Internal temperature will rise 5°F during standing.) Place fruit kabobs on cooking grid. Grill, covered, for 6 to 8 minutes, or until lightly browned, turning over once.

Carve pork diagonally into thin slices. In large mixing bowl or salad bowl, combine pork, fruit and lettuce. In 1-cup measure, combine dressing ingredients. Pour over salad. Toss to coat.

Serving suggestion: Serve with crescent rolls or soft bread sticks.

Per Serving: Calories: 521 • Protein: 28 g. • Carbohydrate: 80 g. • Fat: 13 g. • Cholesterol: 80 mg. • Sodium: 71 mg.
Exchanges: 3 lean meat, 5⅓ fruit, 1 fat

Pork & Peach Salad with Gingered Lime Dressing

Marinade:

¼ cup orange juice
2 tablespoons vegetable oil
1 tablespoon fresh lime juice
½ teaspoon grated fresh gingerroot
⅛ teaspoon crushed red pepper flakes
⅛ teaspoon ground cinnamon
⅛ teaspoon ground cumin

Dressing:

¼ cup orange juice
2 tablespoons vegetable oil
1 tablespoon fresh lime juice
½ teaspoon grated fresh gingerroot
⅛ teaspoon ground cinnamon

1 well-trimmed pork tenderloin (approx. 1 lb.)
2 medium peaches, each cut into 12 wedges

8 cups mixed greens (Bibb lettuce, leaf lettuce, radicchio, escarole and spinach)

4 servings

Serving suggestion: Serve with warm banana muffins.

Per Serving: Calories: 310 • Protein: 28 g. • Carbohydrate: 16 g. • Fat: 16 g. • Cholesterol: 80 mg. • Sodium: 88 mg. Exchanges: 3 lean meat, 2 vegetable, ½ fruit, 1½ fat

How to Make Pork & Peach Salad with Gingered Lime Dressing

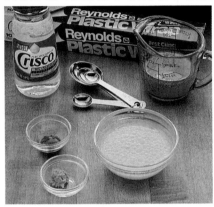

Combine marinade ingredients in small mixing bowl. Microwave at High for 2 to 4 minutes, or until mixture is hot, stirring once. Set aside to cool. In 1-cup measure, combine dressing ingredients. Cover with plastic wrap. Chill.

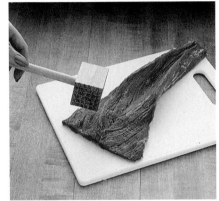

Make horizontal cut through center of tenderloin to within ½ inch of opposite side; do not cut through. Open tenderloin like a book. Pound to an even ½-inch thickness.

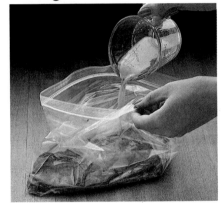

Place meat in large plastic food-storage bag. Add marinade. Secure bag. Turn to coat. Chill 1 to 2 hours, turning bag once or twice. Spray cooking grid with nonstick vegetable cooking spray. Prepare grill for medium direct heat.

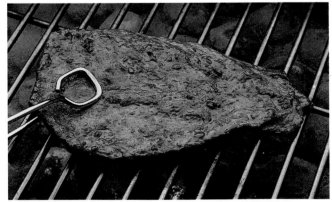

Drain and discard marinade from meat. Place meat on cooking grid. Grill, covered, for 7 to 10 minutes, or until internal temperature registers 160°F and juices run clear. Remove meat from grill. Cover to keep warm.

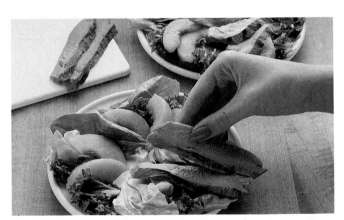

Arrange peach slices and greens evenly on 4 individual serving plates. Carve pork diagonally into thin slices and arrange evenly over greens. Serve with dressing.

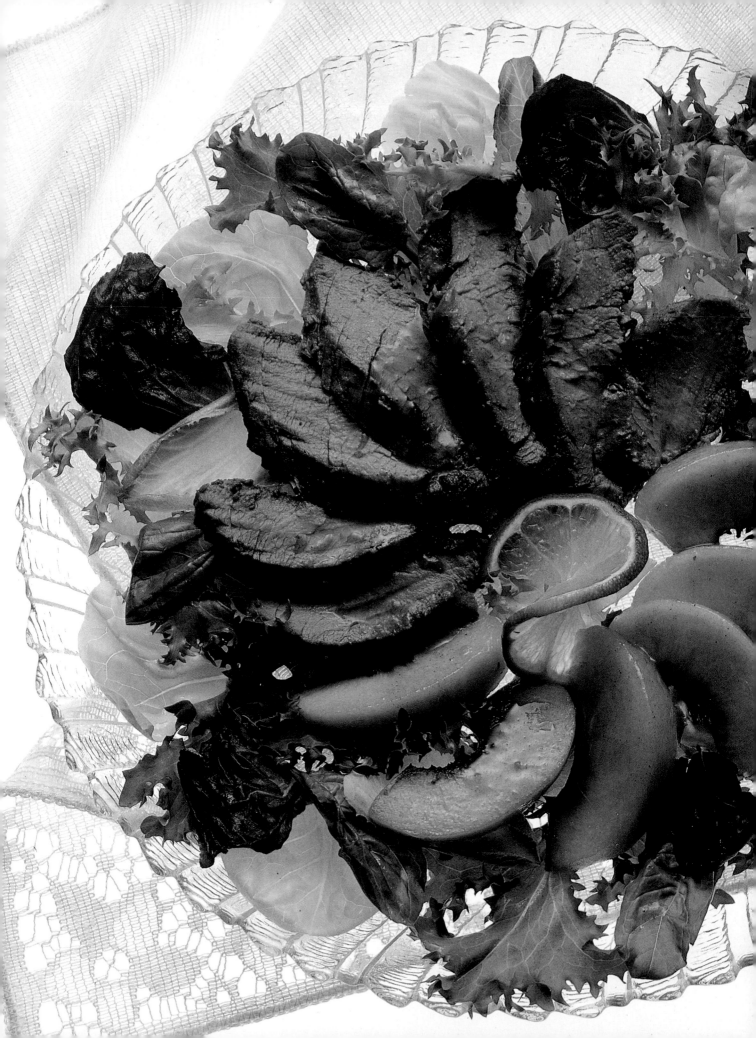

Lamb & Veal

Rosemary & Garlic ▶ Potato Kabobs

16 small new potatoes (about 1 1/2 lbs.)
3 tablespoons water
1 tablespoon olive oil
2 teaspoons snipped fresh rosemary leaves
2 cloves garlic, minced

8 servings

Soak four 10-inch wooden skewers in water for 1/2 hour. Spray cooking grid with nonstick vegetable cooking spray. Prepare grill for medium direct heat.

In 10-inch square or 2-quart casserole, combine potatoes and water. Cover. Microwave at High for 10 to 16 minutes, or until tender, stirring twice. Thread 4 potatoes on each skewer. Place on platter. Set aside.

Combine oil, rosemary and garlic. Brush potatoes evenly with oil mixture. Arrange kabobs on cooking grid. Grill, covered, for 5 to 10 minutes, or until evenly browned, turning over once.

Serving suggestion: Serve with Rosemary Butterflied Leg of Lamb, right.

Per Serving: Calories: 109 • Protein: 2 g.
• Carbohydrate: 21 g. • Fat: 2 g.
• Cholesterol: 0 • Sodium: 9 mg.
Exchanges: 1 1/4 starch, 1/3 fat

Rosemary Butterflied Leg of Lamb ▶

1 1/2 cups port wine
3/4 cup red wine vinegar
1/3 cup olive oil
1 tablespoon plus 1 teaspoon snipped fresh rosemary leaves
8 cloves garlic, minced
4-lb. well-trimmed boneless butterflied lamb leg*

16 servings

In small mixing bowl, combine all ingredients, except lamb. Reserve 3/4 cup marinade. Cover and chill. Place lamb in large plastic food-storage bag. Add remaining marinade. Secure bag. Turn to coat. Chill 2 to 3 hours, turning bag occasionally.

Spray cooking grid with nonstick vegetable cooking spray. Prepare grill for medium indirect heat. Drain and discard marinade from meat. Place lamb over direct heat side of grill to sear for 5 to 8 minutes, or until meat is browned, turning over once. Place lamb cut-side-up over drip pan. Grill, covered, for 45 to 50 minutes, or until desired doneness, basting with reserved marinade every 10 minutes.

Serving suggestion: Serve with Rosemary & Garlic Potato Kabobs, left, and steamed fresh asparagus spears.

Note: Tightly wrap and refrigerate any leftover lamb up to 4 days, or package in freezer containers or bags and freeze 2 to 3 months.

*Order butterflied lamb leg from meat cutter.

Per Serving: Calories: 198 • Protein: 24 g. • Carbohydrate: 2 g. • Fat: 9 g.
• Cholesterol: 76 mg. • Sodium: 59 mg.
Exchanges: 3 lean meat, 1/4 fruit

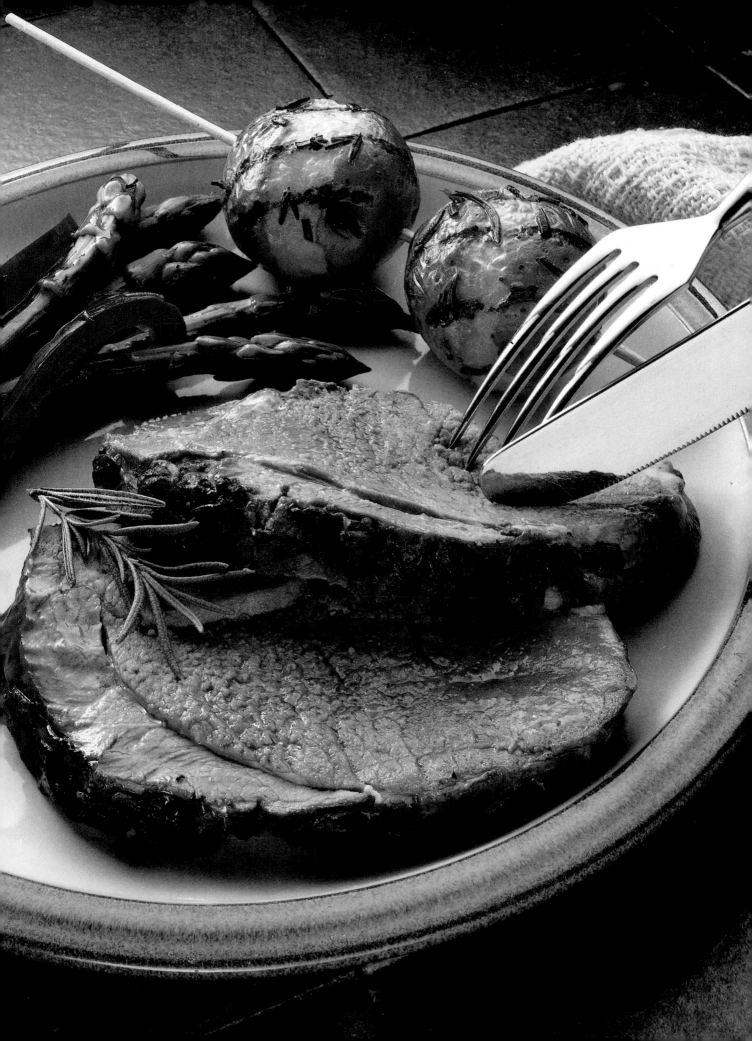

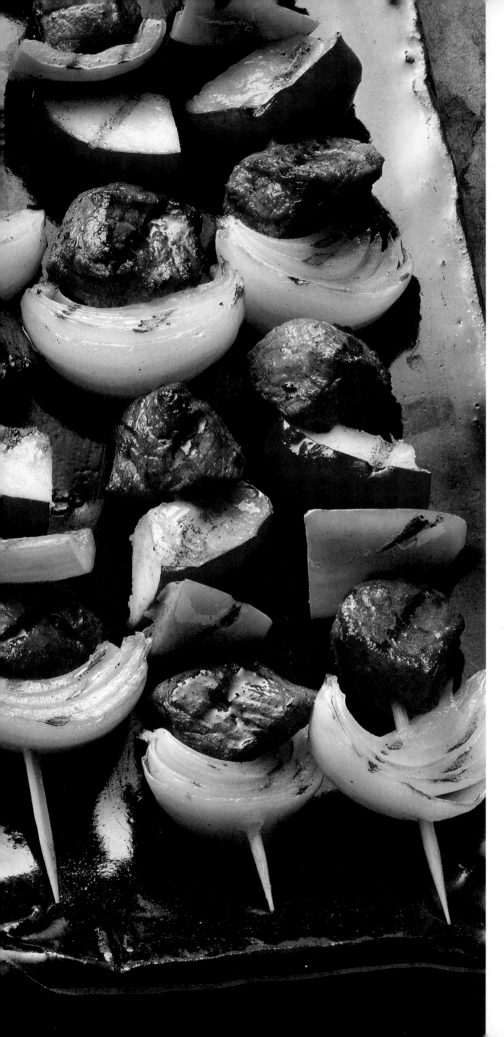

Tandoori Lamb

¼ cup plain nonfat or low-fat
    yogurt
2 tablespoons olive oil,
    divided
1 tablespoon lemon juice
1 tablespoon curry powder
1 clove garlic, minced
1- lb. well-trimmed boneless
    lamb leg, cut into 16 cubes
2 medium onions, each cut
    into 6 wedges
½ large green pepper, cut into
    8 chunks
¼ cup water
½ Rome apple, cored and cut
    into 8 chunks

4 servings

Soak four 12-inch wooden
skewers in water for ½ hour. In
medium mixing bowl, combine
yogurt, 1 tablespoon oil, the
lemon juice, curry powder and
garlic. Add lamb. Toss to coat.
Cover with plastic wrap. Chill 15
to 30 minutes.

Spray cooking grid with nonstick
vegetable cooking spray. Prepare
grill for medium direct heat. In
2-quart casserole, combine
onions, green pepper and water.
Cover. Microwave at High for 4
to 6 minutes, or until onions are
tender-crisp, stirring once. Drain.
Add apple and remaining 1 tablespoon oil. Toss to coat.

Thread each skewer evenly with
onion wedges, lamb cubes and
pepper and apple chunks. Place
kabobs on cooking grid. Grill,
covered, for 12 to 15 minutes, or
until meat is desired doneness,
turning over 2 or 3 times.

Serving suggestion: Serve with
couscous pilaf and Greek salad.

Per Serving: Calories: 268 • Protein: 26 g.
• Carbohydrate: 16 g. • Fat: 11 g.
• Cholesterol: 76 mg. • Sodium: 67 mg.
Exchanges: 3 lean meat, 2½ vegetable,
¼ fruit, ¼ fat

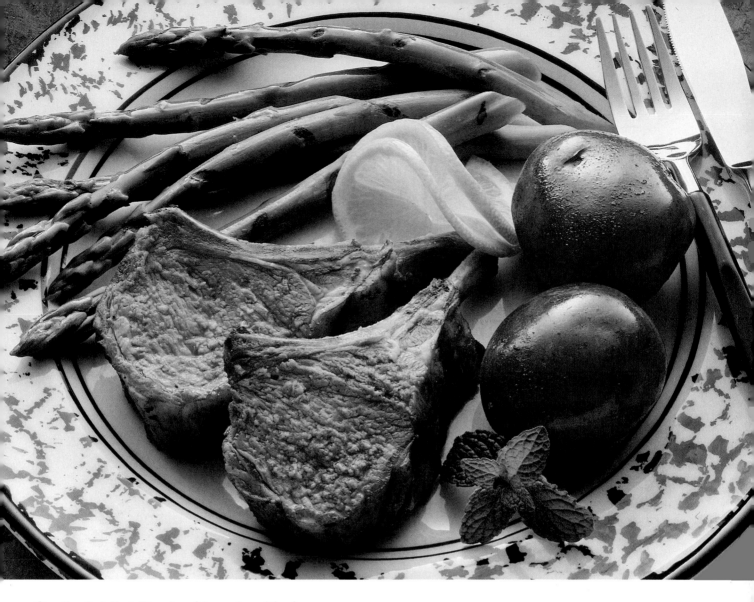

Garlic & Mint Rack of Lamb with Asparagus

1 lb. fresh asparagus
   spears
¼ cup water
¼ cup snipped fresh mint
   leaves
3 tablespoons olive oil, divided
1 tablespoon red wine vinegar
3 cloves garlic, minced
1 teaspoon ground cumin
1 teaspoon cayenne
1 teaspoon salt
1 teaspoon pepper
2 six-rib well-trimmed lamb
   rib rack roasts
   (approximately 1 lb. each)

4 servings

Spray cooking grid with nonstick vegetable cooking spray. Prepare grill for medium direct heat. Arrange asparagus in 8-inch square baking dish. Add water. Cover with plastic wrap. Microwave at High for 5 to 6 minutes, or until asparagus brightens in color, rearranging spears once. Drain. Set aside.

In blender, combine mint, 2 tablespoons oil, the vinegar, garlic, cumin, cayenne, salt and pepper. Process until smooth. Shield bone ends of each lamb rack with foil. Spread mint mixture evenly over exterior meaty surface of each rack. Insert meat thermometer. Place racks bone-sides-up on cooking grid. Grill, covered, for 15 to 18 minutes for rare (135°F) to medium (155°F), or to desired doneness, turning over once. Remove from grill. Let stand, tented with foil, for 10 minutes. (Internal temperature will rise 5°F during standing.)

Brush asparagus with remaining 1 tablespoon oil. Arrange spears crosswise on cooking grid. Grill, covered, for 4 to 5 minutes, or until lightly browned, turning over once.

Serving suggestion: Serve with steamed whole new potatoes.

Per Serving: Calories: 311 • Protein: 24 g. • Carbohydrate: 4 g. • Fat: 22 g.
• Cholesterol: 75 mg. • Sodium: 622 mg.
Exchanges: 3 lean meat, ¾ vegetable, 2¾ fat

151

Grilled Lemon Tarragon Veal & Artichokes ▶

Marinade:

1/4 cup fresh lemon juice
1/4 cup dry white wine
2 tablespoons vegetable oil
2 teaspoons dried tarragon
   leaves
2 teaspoons sugar
1/2 teaspoon grated lemon peel

4 well-trimmed bone-in veal
   rib or loin chops (6 oz. each),
   1/2 inch thick
2 artichokes (about 12 oz.
   each)

4 servings

In 1-cup measure, combine marinade ingredients. Reserve 1/4 cup marinade. Cover and chill. Place veal in large plastic food-storage bag. Add remaining marinade. Secure bag. Turn to coat. Chill 30 minutes, turning once.

Spray cooking grid with nonstick vegetable cooking spray. Prepare grill for medium direct heat. Trim stems of artichokes flush with base. Rinse well. Shake off excess water. Wrap each artichoke in plastic wrap. Microwave at High for 7 to 10 minutes, or until lower leaves can be removed easily and base can be pierced easily with fork, rearranging once. Let stand, wrapped, for 5 minutes. Cut each artichoke in half lengthwise, keeping leaves intact. Scrape out and discard choke. Set aside.

Drain and discard marinade from meat. Place veal on cooking grid. Grill, covered, for 12 to 14 minutes, or just until meat is no longer pink, turning once and basting twice with reserved marinade. During last 5 minutes of grilling veal, place artichoke halves cut-sides-down on cooking grid. Grill, covered, until lightly browned, turning over once and basting twice with reserved marinade.

Serving suggestion: Serve with baked potatoes and fresh fruit salad.

Per Serving: Calories: 238 • Protein: 24 g. • Carbohydrate: 11 g. • Fat: 11 g.
• Cholesterol: 90 mg. • Sodium: 137 mg.
Exchanges: 3 lean meat, 1½ vegetable, ¼ fruit, ½ fat

Orange Herbed Veal Roast with Fruited Wild Rice

Marinade:

2 tablespoons vegetable oil
1 clove garlic, minced
1/2 cup orange juice
1 teaspoon dried sage leaves
1 teaspoon dried thyme
   leaves

3-lb. well-trimmed
   boneless veal loin roast
3¼ cups water, divided
1 cup orange juice
1/2 teaspoon salt
1⅓ cups uncooked wild rice
1/2 teaspoon dried sage leaves
1/2 teaspoon dried thyme leaves
1/2 cup dried apricot halves,
   cut into small pieces
1/2 cup currants
1/4 cup snipped fresh parsley

12 servings

In small mixing bowl, combine oil and garlic. Cover with plastic wrap. Microwave at High for 2 to 3 minutes, or until garlic is tender, stirring once. Add remaining marinade ingredients. Mix well. Place roast in large plastic food-storage bag. Add marinade to bag. Secure bag. Turn to coat. Chill 2 to 4 hours, turning bag occasionally.

Spray cooking grid with nonstick vegetable cooking spray. Prepare grill for medium indirect heat. Place drip pan on empty side of grill. Drain and discard marinade from meat. Insert meat thermometer. Place roast on cooking grid over drip pan. Cover. Grill for 1 hour 15 minutes to 1 hour 30 minutes for medium (155°F) to well (165°F), turning over once. Add additional coals to grill after 1 hour.

Meanwhile, in 3-quart saucepan, combine 3 cups water, the orange juice and salt. Cook conventionally over high heat until mixture begins to boil. Reduce heat to low. Add wild rice, sage and thyme. Cover. Cook for 1 hour to 1 hour 15 minutes, or until rice is tender. Drain (if all liquid is not absorbed). In 2-quart casserole, combine remaining 1/4 cup water and the apricots. Cover. Microwave at High for 4 to 5 minutes, or until apricots are plumped, stirring once. Add wild rice mixture, currants and parsley. Mix well. Let roast stand, tented with foil, for 10 minutes before carving. (Internal temperature will rise 5°F during standing.) Carve roast across grain into thin slices.

Serving suggestion: Serve with lightly buttered Brussels sprouts.

Note: Tightly wrap and refrigerate any leftover veal up to 4 days, or package in freezer containers or bags and freeze 3 months.

Per Serving: Calories: 265 • Protein: 26 g. • Carbohydrate: 24 g. • Fat: 7 g.
• Cholesterol: 90 mg. • Sodium: 176 mg.
Exchanges: 1¼ starch, 3 lean meat, ⅓ fruit

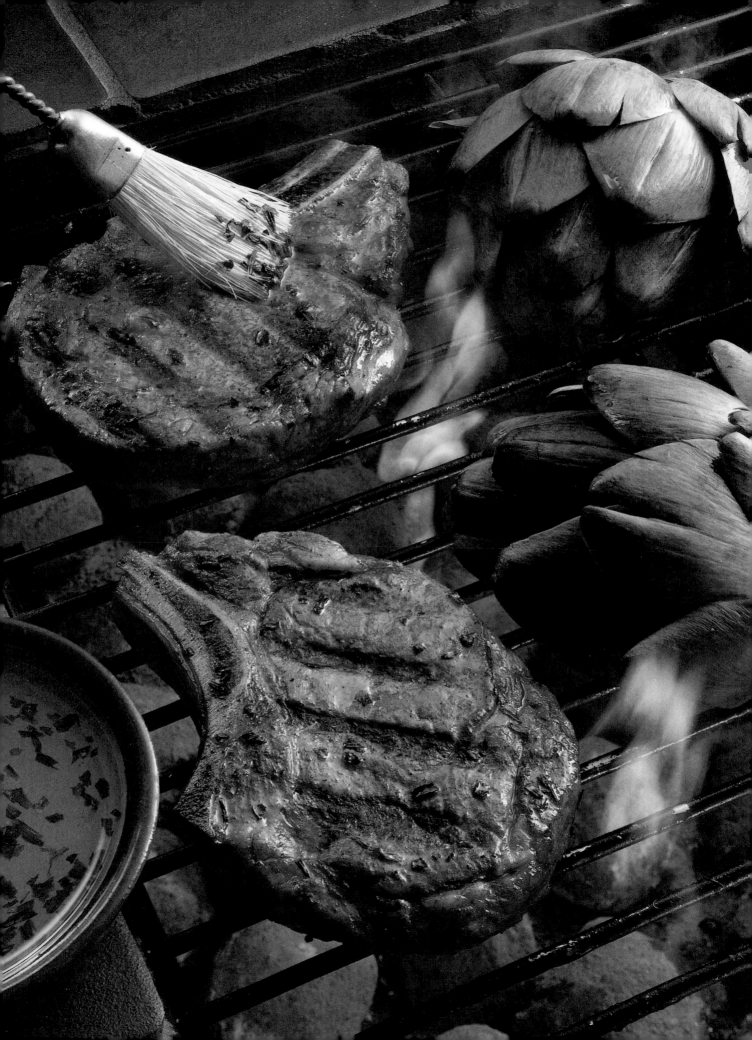

Index

Cy DeCosse Incorporated offers
Microwave Cooking Accessories
at special subscriber discounts.
For information write:

Microwave Accessories
5900 Green Oak Drive
Minnetonka, MN 55343